Neural Control
of Circulation

Research Topics in Physiology

Charles D. Barnes, *Editor*
Department of Physiology
Texas Tech University School of Medicine
Lubbock, Texas

1. Donald G. Davies and Charles D. Barnes (Editors). Regulation of Ventilation and Gas Exchange, 1978

2. Maysie J. Hughes and Charles D. Barnes (Editors). Neural Control of Circulation, 1980

In preparation

3. John Orem and Charles D. Barnes (Editors), Physiology in Sleep, 1981

Neural Control
of Circulation

Edited by

MAYSIE J. HUGHES

CHARLES D. BARNES

Department of Physiology
Texas Tech University
School of Medicine
Lubbock, Texas

1980

ACADEMIC PRESS

A Subsidiary of Harcourt Brace Jovanovich, Publishers

New York   London   Toronto   Sydney   San Francisco

ACADEMIC PRESS, INC.
111 Fifth Avenue, New York, New York 10003

United Kingdom Edition published by
ACADEMIC PRESS, INC. (LONDON) LTD.
24/28 Oval Road, London NW1 7DX

Library of Congress Cataloging in Publication Data

Main entry under title:

Neural control of circulation.

    (Research topics in physiology ;)
    Includes bibliographies and index.
    1. Nervous system, Vasomotor. I. Hughes,
Maysie J. II. Barnes, Charles Dee. III. Series.
[DNLM: 1. Blood circulation. 2. Nervous system
--Physiology. 3. Cardiovascular system--
Innervation. WG103 N494]
QP109.N48   612'.1   79–6784
ISBN 0–12–360850–3

Contents

7. Pharmacological Aspects of Neural Control of the Circulation

Chung Chinn

List of Contributors

Numbers in parentheses indicate the pages on which the authors' contributions begin.

Cliff A. Astley (1), Physiology and Biophysics and Regional Primate Research Center, University of Washington, Seattle, Washington 98195

Chung Chinn * (149), Department of Physiology, Texas Tech University School of Medicine, Lubbock, Texas 79430

E. Costa (103), Laboratory of Preclinical Pharmacology, National Institute of Mental Health, Saint Elizabeths Hospital, Washington, D.C. 20032

Gerard L. Gebber (51), Department of Pharmacology and Toxicology, Michigan State University, East Lansing, Michigan 48824

A. Roger Hohimer † (1), Physiology and Biophysics and Regional Primate Research Center, University of Washington, Seattle, Washington 98195

Raymond C. Koehler (123), Department of Physiology, School of Medicine, State University of New York at Buffalo, Buffalo, New York 14214

John A. Krasney (123), Department of Physiology, School of Medicine, State University of New York at Buffalo, Buffalo, New York 14214

Donald J. Reis (81), Laboratory of Neurobiology, Department of Neurology, Cornell University Medical College, New York, New York 10021

* Present address: Department of Neurosciences, CMDNJ, New Jersey Medical School, East Orange, New Jersey 07018.

† Present address: Department of Obstetrics and Gynecology, University of Oregon Health Sciences Center, Portland, Oregon 97102.

Orville A. Smith (1), Physiology and Biophysics and Regional Primate Research Center, University of Washington, Seattle, Washington 98195

Robert B. Stephenson (1), Physiology and Biophysics and Regional Primate Research Center, University of Washington, Seattle, Washington 98195

Jean C. Strahlendorf (23), Departments of Physiology and Pharmacology, Texas Tech University Health Sciences Center, Lubbock, Texas 79430

Howard K. Strahlendorf (23), Departments of Physiology and Pharmacology, Texas Tech University Health Sciences Center, Lubbock, Texas 79430

Preface

This second volume in the series *Research Topics in Physiology* presents an in-depth view of specialized areas in the neurophysiology of circulation that are currently being intensively investigated. Eminent investigators in specialized subareas here review their own work and place it in perspective. They were charged with presenting the historical basis and theory from which the current research interest evolved, the current status of the field, and directions for future research. Special emphasis was placed on critical evaluation of the experimental data in each scientist's research area.

The neural regulation of the circulatory system is looked at in a comprehensive manner with specific research approaches treated in greater depth. The chapters in this volume begin at the cerebral level and progress downward through the neural axis. The first chapter is a synthesis of the research done in a large number of studies using conscious animals, the results of which have necessitated rethinking the mechanisms of cardiovascular control. The second chapter summarizes the present knowledge of the contribution of the brain stem and cerebellum to cardiovascular control. Next, specific research areas concerning bulbospinal control of sympathetic nerve discharge are discussed. This is followed by a chapter devoted to a particularly active area of research interest, the nucleus tractus solitarii and experimental neurogenic hypertension. Chapter 5 explores a new concept in potential hypertensive mechanisms involving long-term transsynaptic regulation of adrenal medullary function. The neural control of the circulation during hypoxia is treated in Chapter 6 and finally, aspects of central nervous system pharmacology and regulation of circulation are discussed.

This volume is designed for all those individuals who are interested in the cardiovascular system and its function. It is an in-depth presentation of current theoretical and experimental aspects of neural control of circulation, and should prove useful, not only to individuals specifically interested in this field, but to students and researchers in physiology and individuals in other ancillary areas of bioscience. It is the hope of the editors that this book will be provocative and stimulate future research between the areas of cardiovascular- and neurophysiology.

Maysie J. Hughes
Charles D. Barnes

1

Behavioral and Cerebral Control of Cardiovascular Function

Orville A. Smith, Cliff A. Astley,
A. Roger Hohimer, and Robert B. Stephenson

I. INTRODUCTION

In the study of neural regulation of the cardiovascular (CV) system, the complexity of the system increases as you proceed up the neuraxis from spinal cord to cerebrum. Therefore, precise statements about the relation between function and structure become increasingly difficult to make. At the spinal level reflexes can be studied; the size of the fibers on the input side can be identified; and their type can be designated as muscle afferents, cutaneous afferents, tendon and joint afferents, etc.

1

NEURAL CONTROL OF CIRCULATION

One can also determine that the output emanates from a particular sympathetic or parasympathetic segment. Therefore, CV spinal reflexes may be specified as to their adequate stimuli, the route and location of synapses involved, and the function of the reflex. At this spinal level the use of anesthetics does not seem to be a severe drawback in the analysis of function and structure.

This situation changes rapidly at the medulla and the "vasomotor centers," where the number of synapses in the system increases, and even the pathways for the reflexes found at this level are not known. At the level of the diencephalon, where there are no reflexes to be studied and inputs are extremely ambiguous, a host of uncertainties arise. What is being stimulated when electrical current passes through a volume of tissue? What is the function of a particular nucleus or tract? What is the significance of deriving one set of CV responses, as a result of stimulating a structure, and a reversed set of these responses, as a result of changing the type of anesthetic? Finally, at the level of the cerebral cortex one is left with few anatomical projections that are clearly related to autonomic functioning, and even those are the subject of a great deal of speculation. At this cortical level anesthetics exert a major effect, making generalizations extremely tenuous.

Despite these uncertainties, in successively higher neural levels, some regulatory functional relations may be specified. In the spinal preparation a distended urinary bladder reflexly leads to extremely high arterial blood pressure levels. The decerebrate preparation shows a consistent, well-integrated baroreflex in response to arterial pressure alterations. At the thalamic levels a sympathetic cholinergic vasodilator system can be demonstrated in the ventral diencephalon. At cortical levels stimulation of area four leads to increased arterial blood flow in the appropriate limb. Because these kinds of relationships can be demonstrated under closely controlled experimental conditions, we are convinced that we understand the system and are tempted to extrapolate from these facts to explain complex homeostatic adjustments in the intact organism.

Historically, one of the best examples of extrapolation from very simple mechanisms to complex integration was the explanation of how the CV response to exercise is regulated. The intrinsic capability of heart muscle to increase its force of contraction as a function of the degree of stretch of the muscle (Starling's law) was stipulated as an essential factor in explaining the increased cardiac output during exercise. Specifically, it was postulated that actively contracting skeletal muscle would act as a peripheral venous pump, resulting in an increased return of venous blood to the heart. This increased return would then increase the filling of the heart, increase heart size, and stretch the heart muscle, which would then contract more vigorously, thereby increasing stroke volume and cardiac output. Most of the mechanisms specified in this scheme were derived from experiments using anesthetized animals or isolated heart preparations and extrapolated to exercising humans. Dr. Robert F. Rushmer (1955; Rushmer and Smith, 1959) created some consternation when, instead of accepting the extrapolation of the results from anesthetized animals, he decided to measure heart size in awake, exercising animals. He found that, during exercise, heart size did not increase; it either decreased or stayed the same. It soon became apparent that the increased stroke volume during exercise was due to neurohumoral factors influencing the force of cardiac contraction, which were not in operation in the anesthetized animal, i.e., control mechanisms derived from a higher level.

Whereas Rushmer's observation does not deny the reality nor the validity of Starling's law of the heart, it does indicate that simply because a mechanism can be shown to exist under experimental conditions, it does not necessarily follow that it will be a major regulatory mechanism or even that it will be used during a particular integrated CV adjustment. Korner (1971) made the point elegantly when he said that attempting to explain complex responses on the basis of action of single variables is unproductive. The danger in attributing control found at one level to the overall regulation, when other higher levels become active, is apparent. Indeed, referring to the examples presented earlier, elevated urinary bladder pressures in the intact organism do not result in excessive arterial pressures; in the intact organism the baroreflex is significantly altered by the behavior of the organism at that time; the functional significance of a sympathetic cholinergic vasodilator system has not yet been specified in the intact organism; and the motor cortex can be removed with no discernible effect on the muscle blood flow changes accompanying exercise.

In summary the attempt to specify the cerebral level of control of the CV system is impeded by two major factors.

1. Anesthetics cannot be used because they exert their major effects directly on the essential anatomical structures that characterize the cerebral cortex and other cerebral structures, i.e., the multiple synapses.

2. There is little understanding of how one level of the central nervous system interacts with the control mechanisms shown to exist at another level.

These factors require that the unanesthetized, normally behaving animal be used to study the cerebral level of CV control, thereby creating a "Catch-22" situation which makes study of the cerebral level nearly impossible. In an unanesthetized animal, all levels of regulation are in operation, so that one ends up studying not only cerebral mechanisms, but the total integrated response with potential contributions from all levels, local as well as neural. Thus, the question regarding what influence cerebral mechanisms have on CV control necessarily becomes more basic: "What are the regulatory mechanisms actually used by the organism in adjusting its circulatory responses to the stresses imposed by the environment and the organism's behavior?" This question must be addressed first if we are ever to approach the question of cerebral control.

This chapter relates efforts to develop a chronic, behaviorally controlled nonhuman primate preparation in which enough important CV variables are measured to enable us to address the rephrased question. With this approach, we hope that some understanding of the role of cerebral mechanisms in CV control eventually may be generated.

II. THE AWAKE, BEHAVIORALLY CONTROLLED PRIMATE PREPARATION

A. Subjects

Juvenile male baboons (*Papio cynocephalus*) weighing 10–15 kg are selected because their size makes implantation of gauges easier, their intelligence makes training easier, and their general physical hardiness increases the probabilities of success.

B. Apparatus and Training

After 2–3 weeks of adaptation to adjustable, three-tiered primate restraint chairs, the baboons are placed for 2–4 hr each day in a ventilated, sound attenuating chamber (1 × 1 × 2 m). The chamber is illuminated by a 60 W overhead white light. A small lamp illuminates the animals' legs. The animals are continuously observed via closed circuit television with one camera focused on the head and one on the legs. External sounds are masked by 60 dB of white noise introduced through a small speaker in the upper corner of the chamber.

The animals are fed sufficient Purina monkey chow to maintain but not gain weight (averaging 140 g chow per day); this constitutes mild food deprivation. Feeding is always in the late afternoon after training or testing is completed for the day. The animals are weighed daily to check their nutritional state.

Three easily visible and different colored stimulus lights are placed

in front of the animal to signal which behavior, if any, is to be reinforced. Reinforcements of 0.6 ml of applesauce are delivered via a feeder
tube.

After at least 1 week of adaptation to the chamber, the animals are
trained using operant techniques to perform 4 min of mild dynamic leg
exercise on a wheel with an adjustable brake. The wheel is positioned
so that it is easily within reach of the baboon's feet. Initially, reinforcements are delivered in the presence of a particular stimulus light with
no response required of the animal; this training establishes a relation
between the stimulus and the availability of food reward. Subsequently,
the light is turned on, but the animal is rewarded only when he touches
the exercise wheel and later only when he turns the wheel. This training
is accomplished over 2–5 weeks.

The baboons are then trained to press a small lever with one hand.
Again, the standard operant technique of successive approximation is
used and a different light signals the lever press condition. After the
animal associates the lever press with reinforcement, the number of lever
presses per reinforcement is increased by randomizing the time interval
between reinforcements. Eventually the baboons press at constant rates
and are rewarded about once every 15 sec.

After the lever press and exercise behaviors are stabilized, the procedures for the conditioned emotional response (CER) are started. A
conditioning trial consists of turning on a conditioned stimulus (CS),
an auditory signal ("Sonalert," 2900 Hz, 80 dB interrupted 2.5 times
per second), for 1 min and terminating it simultaneously with the unconditioned stimulus (UCS)—a 1 or 2 sec, 10 to 15 mA shock delivered
through clips placed on the skin of the abdomen. Only one trial is given
during any one-day training session, and one or two days elapse between
each trial. Each animal is given 10–12 trials.

In addition to these active behaviors, the CV responses to passive behaviors are obtained while the animal sits quietly between sessions ("rest"
condition), while it consumes applesauce automatically delivered without requiring a task of the animal ("eating" condition), and during the
middle of the night when observations via the closed circuit television
indicate that the baboon is asleep ("sleep" condition).

C. Surgery

After training is completed, aseptic surgery is performed under halothane anesthesia. A silastic-covered, polyvinyl chloride cannula is implanted in the left axillary artery and channeled subcutaneously to the
abdominal region where it exits the skin. Patency is maintained by con-

tinuous infusion of heparinized saline (2–5 U/ml, 100 ml per day). A ventral midline transperitoneal approach is used to place a 3–3.5 mm electromagnetic flow transducer (Zepeda Instruments, Seattle) and a silastic occluder around the left renal artery, taking care not to damage the renal nerves; a 6 mm transducer and silastic occluder are placed around the terminal aorta. The lead wires to the flow transducer and the occluder tubes exit the body wall and skin at the umbilical level. The animals are then dressed in short-sleeved nylon jackets with skirts that are secured to the middle plastic tier of the chair to keep the animals from reaching the lead wires and tubes. The animals recover for 1 week before training is resumed and at least 3 weeks before data are collected.

D. Instrumentation

A transparent plastic dome that covers the baboon's head is used to collect expired gas; 15 liters/min of air are withdrawn from the top of the dome while air inflow is allowed only through the small gaps between the animal's neck and the top level of the chair. Oxygen consumption ($\dot{V}_{O_2}$) is estimated as the product of air flow rate and the difference in oxygen fraction between the ambient chamber air and that being withdrawn from the hood. Flow is measured with an anemometer (Thermosystems, Inc., St. Paul, MN, model 1054B) and oxygen fraction with an oxygen cell (Thermox I analyzer, Thermo-Lab, Pittsburg, PA). Oxygen consumption is corrected to STPD. Calibrations are made with room air and two standard gases of known O_2 content. Arterial blood pressure is measured from the axillary cannula with a pressure transducer (Statham, Oxnard, CA, model P23dB) referenced to heart level and calibrated with a standard mercury manometer. Heart rate is derived via a cardiotachometer (Beckman, Schiller Park, IL, type 9867B) triggered from the blood pressure pulse. Blood flow transducers are connected to appropriate drivers and amplifiers (Zepeda Instruments, Seattle). Zero flow is determined by inflating the occluder placed around the vessel distal to the proble. *In vivo* sensitivity of the flow measurement system is determined as described by Astley *et al.* (1979). All physiologic data are recorded on Offner eight-channel recorders.

E. Experimental Sequence

The baboon is transported from the animal quarters and weighed enroute to the experimental chamber. When measurements of $\dot{V}_{O_2}$ are desired, the plastic dome is placed over the baboon's head and attached to the chair, and the applesauce delivery tube is introduced through the front of the dome. The animal is then placed in the sound attenuating chamber, the transducers and electrodes are attached, and the chamber door is closed. Instruments are calibrated before and after each session.

The animals are in the chamber for 15–30 min before the first stimulus is introduced. This first stimulus is usually the signal for exercise, which continues for 4 min. After a recovery period of 5–15 min, the next condition is initiated, which usually is the signal for lever press; this also proceeds for 4 min. After another recovery period, the next condition begins—either free-feeding, a repeat of exercise or lever press, or the CER if it is scheduled for that day.

The procedure for the CER is begun by presenting the visual signal for the lever press condition. After at least 1 min of stable lever pressing, the CS signal is introduced for 60 sec. The signal then goes off and the UCS is delivered. The signal for lever press remains on during presentation of the CS and for another 3 min after the UCS. A recovery period of 5–15 min ensues and then one of the other behavioral conditions is repeated.

During any one experimental day, each session of lever press, exercise, and free-feed is presented two to four times. The CER condition is introduced only every second or third day, and only once each day. The variability of stimulus presentation and time intervals prevents the animal from learning a pattern or anticipating the next stimulus to be presented.

Records during sleep are obtained by leaving the baboon in the chamber overnight and sampling several times during the night.

F. Data Collection and Analysis

Sessions are accepted for analysis only if behaviors are relatively continuous, if vessel occlusion gives reliable flow zero, and if there is no evidence of cross-flow transducer interaction. Instantaneous signals from the transducers are recorded on strip chart recorders, digitally sampled at 100 Hz, and averaged in 3-sec bins using a laboratory computer (Digital Equipment, Inc., Maynard, MA, model PDP-8/E). Renal and terminal aortic vascular resistances are computed digitally. The automatic data collection format is 1 min of resting control, then 4 min of exercise, feeding, or lever pressing followed by 3 min of recovery. In the CER condition, 1 min of baseline lever pressing, 1 min of CS signal, and 3 min of recovery are recorded. Multiple runs of a particular behavior from one animal are averaged digitally and plotted with a graphics printer (Versatec, Inc., Santa Clara, CA, model D1100 printer/plotter).

After enough trials of each behavior are obtained, so that the average response is stable and has a low variability, one or more of the experimental manipulations are performed.

III. RESULTS

An example of the CV response accompanying each kind of behavior being studied is presented in Figs. 1–5. These are the analog records of one response from one animal. A great deal of variability might be expected from a single record; however, because of the precise environmental control and the extended training periods, the individual responses from one session to another and even from one animal to the next are much the same. This can be observed by comparing the pattern of these responses with those in Figs. 6 and 7, which are the computer averages of the mean responses of five trials on each of six or seven animals. Figures 6 and 7 also present the patterns of vascular-bed resistance changes derived from the computer analysis.

The largest changes occur, as expected, with exercise and emotion. The rapid increase in heart rate, blood pressure, and terminal

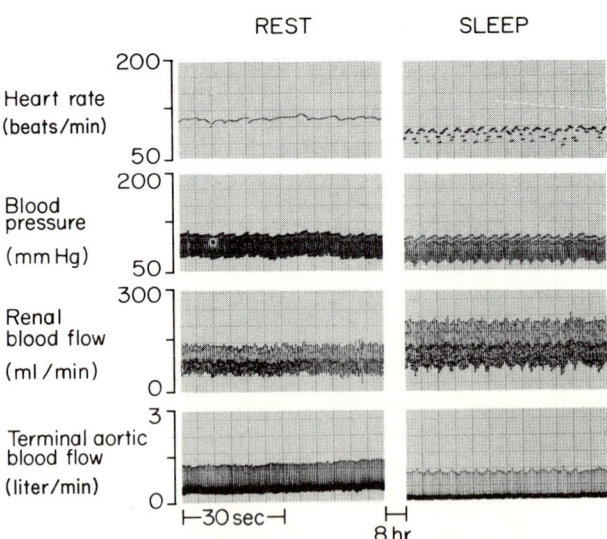

Fig. 1. Comparison of CV variables during sleep and quiet, awake rest.

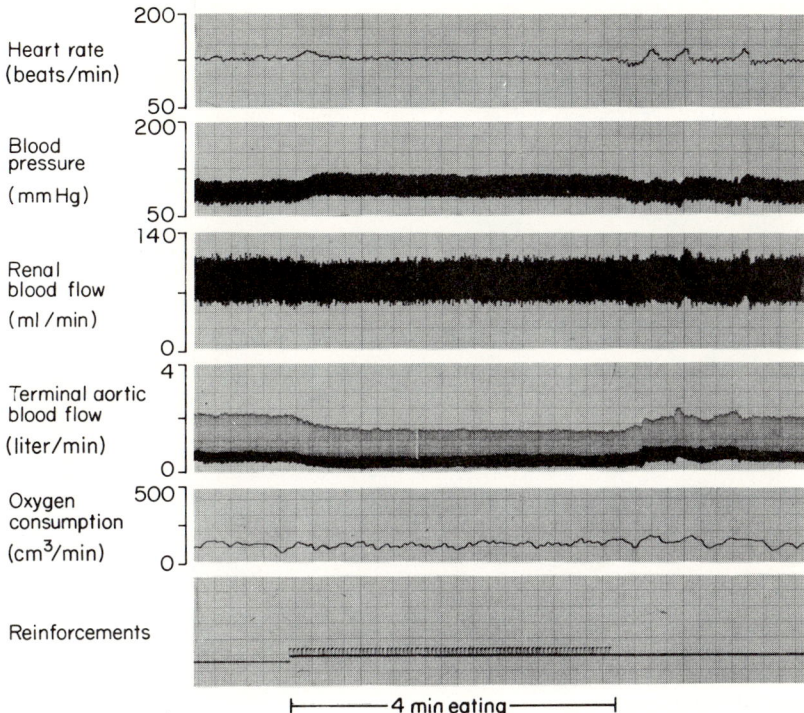

Fig. 2. CV responses to ingesting periodically delivered applesauce (0.6 ml at a time).

aortic flow followed by slower changes in renal resistance, $\dot{V}_{O_2}$, and further heart rate and pressure response during exercise are shown in Fig. 6. Figure 7 demonstrates the characteristic multiphasic CV responses accompanying the emotional situation. Although not as dramatic, the small, systematic changes that occur during eating and lever press also hold promise for interesting functional analysis. The remarkable increase in terminal aortic resistance during eating is unexpected and suggests the elicitation of a fairly powerful reflex during eating which actively constricts hindlimb beds.

We have begun to analyze some of the mechanisms controlling these normal responses. While investigating the renal response to exercise, Hohimer and Smith (1979) found that, during the last minute of exercise, blood flow through the normal renal artery was decreased $20 \pm 3\%$ (SEM) with respect to blood flow during the minute of rest preceding the exercise. This response occurred within 1.5 min, was

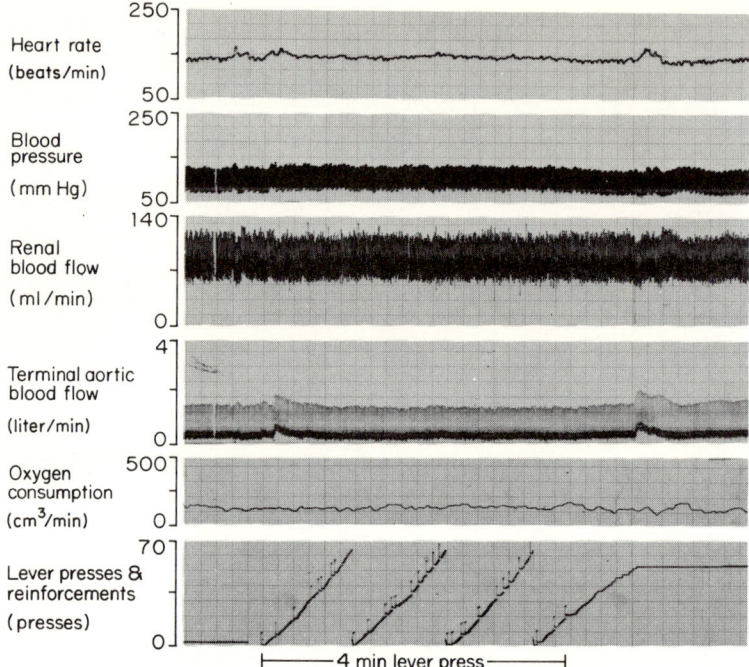

Fig. 3.   CV changes accompanying lever pressing for a food reward.

maintained throughout the exercise, and recovered to control within 2 min. Mean arterial blood pressure rose $21 \pm 2\%$, renal vascular resistance rose $46 \pm 6\%$, heart rate rose $42 \pm 3.9\%$, and $\dot{V}_{O_2}$ increased from 6.2 to 20.2 cm³ O_2/kg/min. Behavioral situations simulating the arousal and feeding components of the exercise task, but not requiring muscular exertion, did not alter renal blood flow (RBF). In four of the animals, blood flow to the contralateral but surgically denervated kidney was measured; it increased transiently at the onset of exercise but returned to control by the last minute of work. Thus, the baboon, like man, shows a decrease in RBF during exercise. This response has a rapid onset and recovery and is primarily neurally mediated.

In another study, we analyzed the responses during the reproducible elicitation of a CER (Smith *et al.*, 1979). Sections of renal nerves and autonomic pharmacologic interventions were used to determine the mechanisms for the CV responses accompanying the CER. The resistance changes in the renal and hindlimb vascular beds were generated by rapid, neurally mediated vasoconstriction of the renal vasculature; and by a slower acting, circulating vasoactive agent, probably epinephrine,

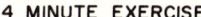

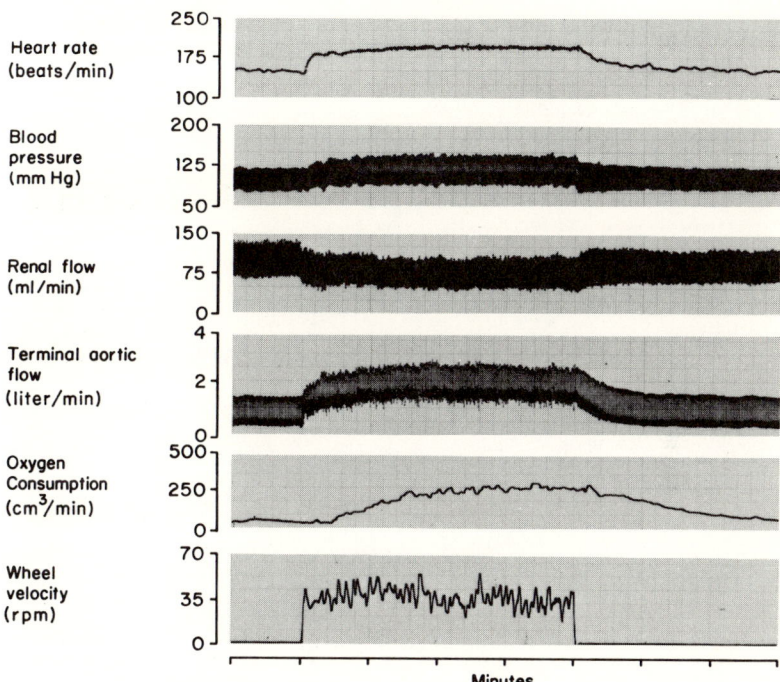

Fig. 4. CV responses accompanying 4 min of moderate exercise.

which causes a delayed second constriction in the renal bed and a net dilation in the hindlimbs.

The occluder on the terminal aorta, which is used to determine flow zero, can also be used to provide a square wave increase in arterial pressure by sudden inflation of the cuff. The arterial baroreceptors then respond to this change, and a baroreflex is elicited whenever desired. Figure 8 illustrates a baroreflex imposed on five behavioral situations. These data suggest that the type of behavior affects the relation between the amount of pressure increase and the amount of heart rate decrease, i.e., the sensitivity (or gain) is changed. We have analyzed this relationship more precisely (Stephenson and Smith, 1977; Stephenson *et al.*, 1975), using a modification of the preparation described above. We studied neural regulation of heart rate in baboons during sleep, lever press for food reinforcement, eating, and mild dynamic leg exercise. Propranolol decreased blood pressure and heart rate during exercise, but had little effect during the other behaviors, while atropine elevated pressure and rate during all behaviors except exercise. In the normal situation then,

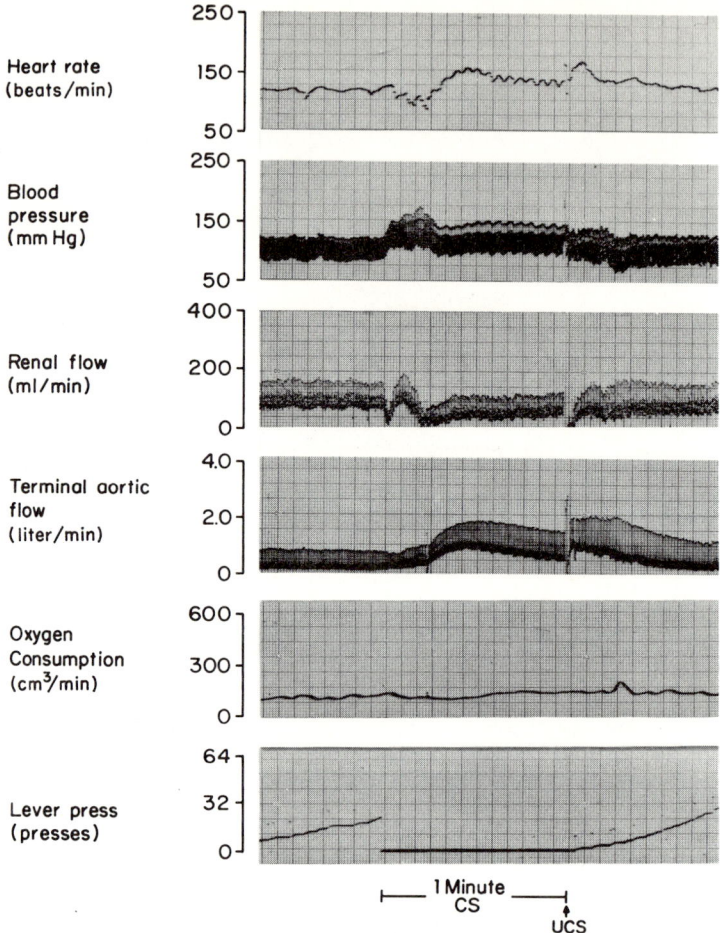

Fig. 5. CV response to a conditioned emotional response.

sympathetic tone is high and vagal tone is low during exercise, while the opposite holds during the other behaviors. Reflex control of heart rate was studied by forcing blood pressure sinusoidally by inflating and deflating a cuff placed around the descending aorta (instead of the terminal aorta). Reflex sensitivity determined by either heart rate, heart interval, or proportional change was highest during sleep and lowest during exercise. Propranolol had little effect on sensitivity, but atropine reduced sensitivity to low levels during all behaviors. The sympathetic contribution to the baroreflex was small at all times; the vagal contribution was large during sleep, smaller during lever press and eating, and smallest during exercise. Reflex time lag was long during exercise (de-

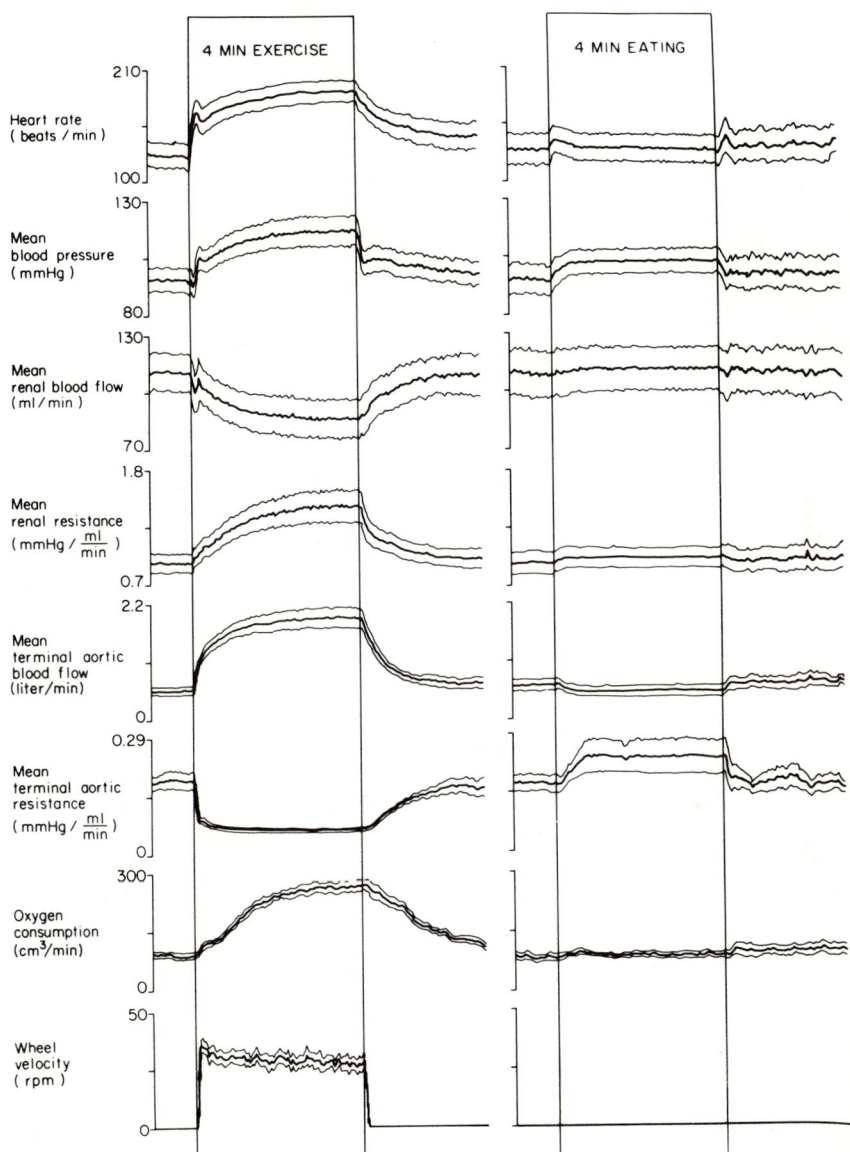

Fig. 6. Averaged CV response during exercise and eating ($n = 7$). Dark line = mean, light line = 1 standard error.

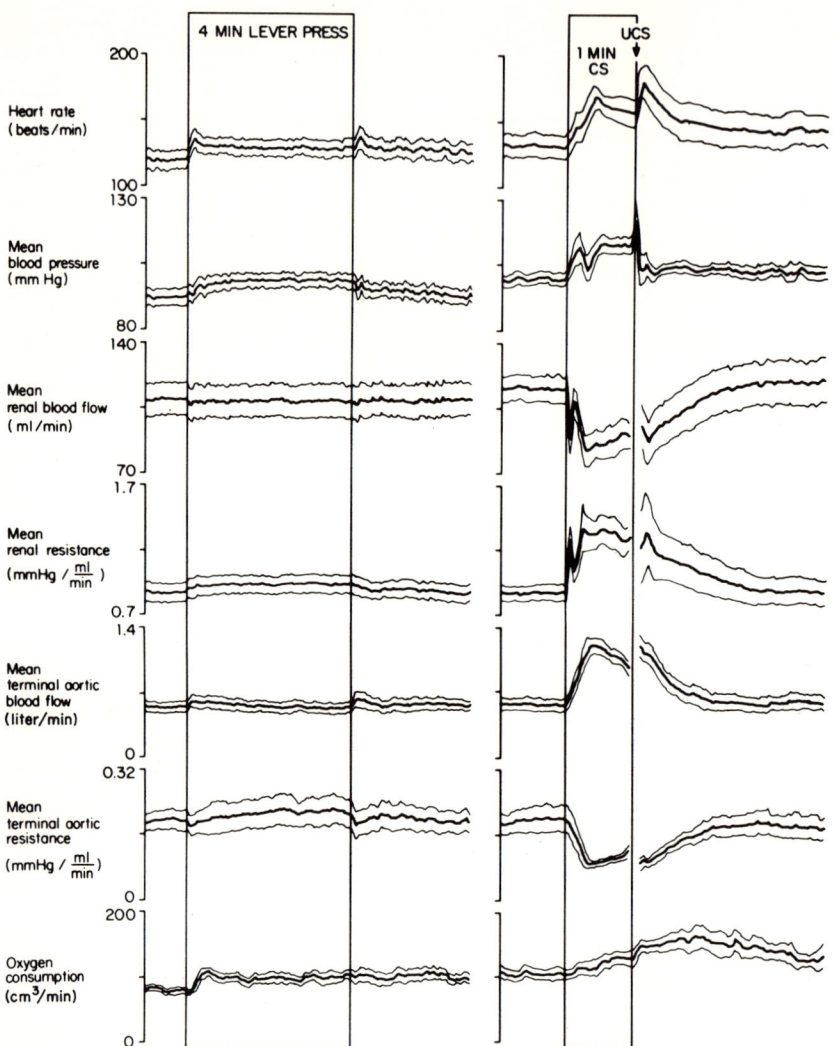

Fig. 7. Averaged CV response during lever press $(n = 7)$ and CER $(n = 6)$. Dark line = mean. Light line = 1 standard error.

noting sympathetic dominance) and short during the other behaviors (denoting vagal dominance). It was concluded that the differences in baroreflex sensitivity among behaviors are mediated by central neural modulation of the vagal component of the reflex.

Because we can measure CV variables at any time of the day or night during any well controlled or freely occurring behavior, we can look at relations between variables in a way not commonly done. It is, in

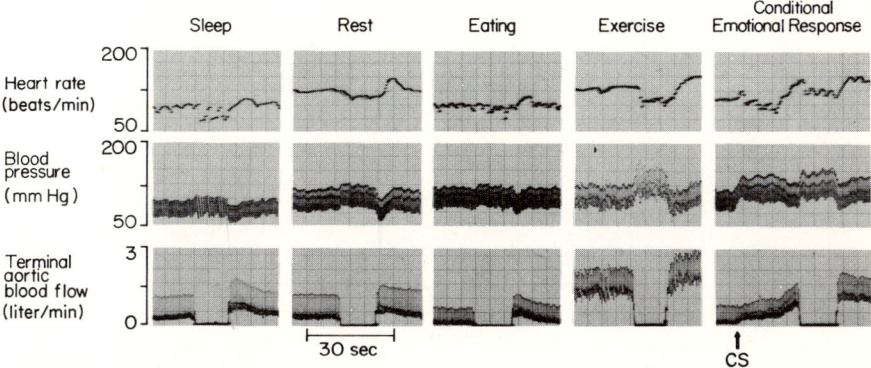

Fig. 8. Effect of sudden occlusion of blood flow through the terminal aorta on blood pressure and reflex heart changes. Influence of behavior on the magnitude of the bradycardia is seen in the first 3 panels (similar pressure increases but different heart rate changes). The last 2 panels show larger pressure changes with bradycardia, similar to a sleep situation.

effect, a means of allowing the most natural experiments to occur while the observer simply collects the information. The relation between mean renal blood flow and mean arterial pressure has been examined by averaging the values of these variables during the last 0.5 or 1 min of a stable behavior, e.g., the average value of mean flow and mean pressure was determined for the last minute of the 4-min exercise period. For the CER, which lasts only 1 min, the value of the last 0.5 min was taken. The point here is that transient responses were excluded; only stabilized response levels were accepted for analysis. This was done for five behaviors ranging from sleep to emotion. In another analysis, the same approach was used to examine heart rate and mean arterial pressure relationships across these same behaviors. The results of these analyses provide some reason to restrict the generality of two of the most fundamental and firmly accepted principles of CV regulation: (1) autoregulation of renal blood flow; and (2) the inverse relation between blood pressure and heart rate.

The classic laboratory experiment to determine the amount of renal blood flow as a function of changing mean blood pressure produces the relationship shown in Fig. 9. The plateau over the range of normal blood pressure (i.e., 80–150 mm Hg) is attributed to an autoregulatory process in the kidney and is commonly used as an example of the "wisdom of the body." The body seemingly provides a constant blood supply to this important organ in spite of major shifts in blood pressure and concomitant alterations of blood supply to other organs during periods of stress. If, however, an animal is allowed to set the blood pressure level by its own behavior, the ensuing relationship between arterial

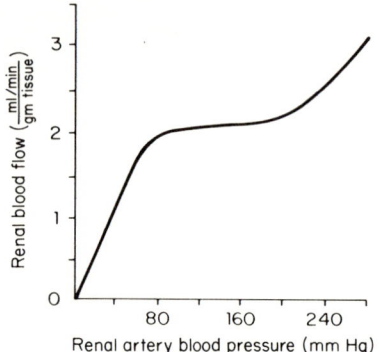

Fig. 9. Renal blood flow as a function of the perfusing arterial blood pressure. Autoregulation is shown between 80 and 200 mm Hg. Anesthetized, artificially perfused preparation.

pressure and mean renal flow is very different. Figure 10 demonstrates that during normal behavior in an awake animal, an inverse relation exists between these variables, which seems contrary to the principle of renal autoregulation. This exists when the nervous system is free to set the levels of these variables.

In a parallel manner, if the classic laboratory preparation (anesthetized, with isolated carotid sinus) is used to alter the mean arterial pressure at the carotid sinus, and the interval between heart beats is plotted against increasing mean pressure, a sigmoid curve [Koch curve (Koch,

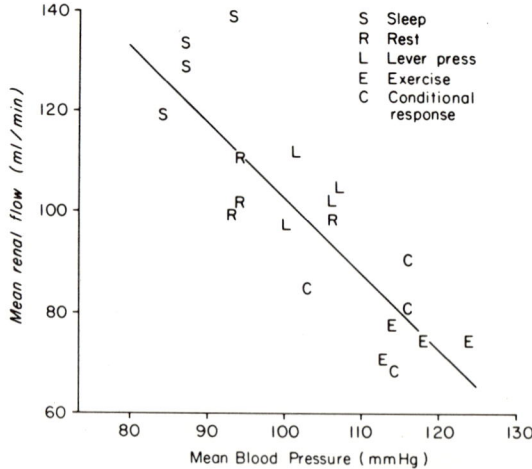

Fig. 10. Relationship of renal flow to blood pressure during 5 behaviors. Responses of 4 animals are presented.

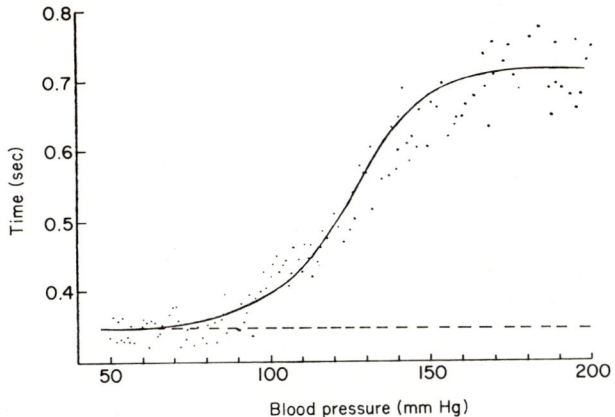

Fig. 11. Relationship of heart interval to mean blood pressure in anesthetized preparation (from Koch, 1931).

1931)] is obtained as in Fig. 11. If the unanesthetized, intact baboon is allowed to set its own mean pressure level by its behavior, the result shown in Fig. 12 is obtained. The data in Figs. 11 and 12 dramatically illustrate the different conclusions obtainable, depending on whether the animal is intact and by what method the independent variable is set. When the higher levels of neural control are allowed to function, the relations between variables may be drastically altered.

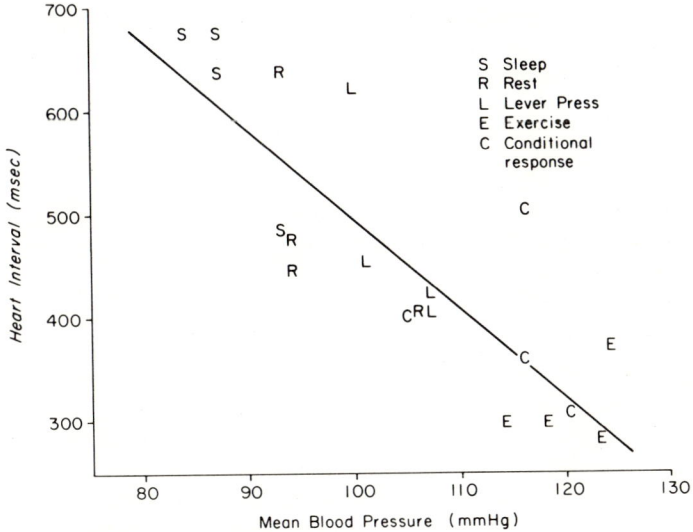

Fig. 12. Relationship of heart interval and mean blood pressure during 5 behaviors. Responses of 4 animals are presented.

IV. DISCUSSION

The point has been made that, in order to study cerebral mechanisms of CV control, it is inappropriate to use anything other than the un-anesthetized, behaviorally controlled preparation in which long-term, repeated measurements of the variables can be made. Also, because of the inherent variability of the autonomic nervous system, these measurements need to be made in many individuals so that the biologic generality of the patterns of response can be assessed.

In achieving this degree of control and measurement capability, it becomes obvious that it is not really the cerebral level of control that is being studied, but rather the total, integrated response involving all levels of control. Indeed, studying the cerebral level of control in isolation becomes a logical impossibility. On this basis, the important question now becomes: "What are the control mechanisms that the *organism actually makes use of* in regulating its CV system?" This is contrasted with the earlier question regarding CV regulation: "What mechanisms exist that in some way influence CV regulation?" This question of biological utility becomes more complex when one recognizes that even though a control mechanism is of critical importance to regulation during a specific stress (behavior or other perturbation), that particular control mechanism may have little or no importance when the stress is from a different source (another behavior).

If this hypothesized dynamic interplay of stresses and control mechanisms is representative of the true situation in the intact organism, then the kind of information presented in Section III becomes important for analyzing and understanding CV control. First, there must be a precise, accurate description of the responses resulting from a given stressor, perturbation, behavior, etc., which causes the CV output to change. Descriptive studies are too frequently passed off as pedestrian or unsophisticated science, while in reality good descriptive studies are too infrequently encountered, even though they provide the essential basis for analysis. Once a response has been described for a particular behavior—using "behavior" generically for any environmental situation resulting in a CV change—(Figs. 1–5) then the generality of that response for the species must be determined (Figs. 6 and 7). At that point, the analysis of mechanisms may begin by devising behavioral, chemical, surgical, mechanical, electronic, or other means of removing or manipulating, in unique fashion, the various control mechanisms potentially responsible for producing the changes associated with this particular behavior. Several studies in our laboratory have demonstrated that the technology is available to carry out controlled experiments in awake, behaving animals and to determine what the biologically significant control mechanisms are in those situations (Hohimer and Smith, 1979; Smith *et al.*, 1979; Stephenson and Smith, 1977).

A major thesis of this chapter is illustrated by the data in Figs. 10 and 11. Keeping Korner's (1971) admonition in mind about single variable explanations of control, it is still difficult to believe that mechanisms as important as renal autoregulation and the baroreflex will not exert a major influence in integrated regulation. However, the data show very clearly that, not only does renal blood flow vary over a wide range of pressures when pressure differences are produced as a concomitant of changing behavior, it actually goes in the opposite direction of expected, normal pressure–flow relations. It is also clear that across these same behaviors there is an *inverse* instead of a direct relation between heart interval and mean arterial pressure. It is true that if one artificially manipulates blood pressure in awake animals, renal autoregulation is still present, as a response to that manipulation (Gross *et al.*, 1976). It can also be shown that if pressure is artificially manipulated during a given behavior (Smyth *et al.*, 1969), the heart interval will be directly related to the pressure level. The biological reality of renal autoregulation and the baroreflex is not in question; they can be demonstrated to exist and to function well in the unanesthetized situation. However, the critical point is that, in order to demonstrate these two principles, pressure has to be changed artificially. In the integrated, freely acting situation, whenever the nervous system brings about a behavioral change that includes a change in pressure, it also acts directly to change renal blood flow or heart interval; it changes them so much that it produces a result *opposite* to the effect expected from the action of autoregulation or the baroreflex in isolation. When confronted with these facts, the CV physiologist says that the animal has shifted from one "state" to another and that the system has been reset to another level, or that a different operating point has been established. However, "resetting" just describes the phenomenon; it does not account for the mechanism by which expected relationships are reversed.

An additional discrepancy appears on closer analysis: the Koch curve (Fig. 11) shows that at mean pressure levels of 80–90 mm Hg, the reflex should be very insensitive, i.e., the slope of the curve is minimal. At pressure levels of 120–130 mm Hg, the sensitivity of the reflex should be maximal, i.e., the slope of the curve is steep. However, the results of Stephenson *et al.* (1975) [with support from the study of Smyth *et al.* (1969)] indicate that during sleep, when low mean-pressure levels of 80–90 mm Hg are found naturally, the reflex sensitivity is maximal. During exercise, when normal pressure levels are 120–130 mm Hg, the reflex sensitivity is at its minimum. It is striking then that in the unanesthetized preparation, not only are the relationships between pressure and rate backward, compared with the anesthetized situation, but the reflex sensitivity bears a far different relation to prevailing blood pressure than would be predicted by the slope of the Koch curve.

In the foregoing, a decided bias has crept into the discourse. The bias is that the cerebral level or at least a "higher level" of the nervous system is responsible for these generally unexpected results. In the strict sense, all that is known is that these differences arise as a concomitant of the total behavior of the organism and are undoubtedly a function of the interaction of many control mechanisms from many sources (Korner, 1971). However, this bias stems from the Hohimer and Smith (1979), Smith *et al.* (1979), and Stephenson and Smith (1977) studies showing the major influence exerted by the nervous system in the determination of what the net outcome of the circulatory response will be.

Acknowledging a bias, it would still seem probable that here we have two excellent examples where higher neural regulation (possibly from the cerebral level) influences and overrides control mechanisms acting at a lower level. Only in situations where pressure changes were produced by some means other than altering integrated higher neural activity, will the lower level mechanisms manifest themselves. This may be what happens in hemorrhage, or possibly with passive postural changes (tilt tables, etc.). Other examples might be found during disease processes. But one rapidly becomes hard pressed to find instances where a behavioral change and the corresponding change in neural activity is not a dominant response to a stress requiring a cardiovascular adjustment. Indeed, these data serve to reopen the question of just how and when the very powerful reflex and local control mechanisms are used. They *must* be very important, but we obviously still do not understand their role in integrated CV adjustments.

Whether the control represented here really emanates from cerebral levels is currently a moot question. Because an organism cannot perform the behaviors without a functional cerebrum, one may assert that the CV control is either equally cerebral or that it simply is unknowable.

ACKNOWLEDGMENTS

We gratefully acknowledge the technical assistance of David J. Taylor and the personnel of the Bioengineering Division of the Regional Primate Research Center. This work was supported by NIH grants HL16910 and RR00166.

REFERENCES

Astley, C. A., Hohimer, A. R., Stephenson, R. B., Smith, O. A., and Spelman, F. A. (1979). Effect of implant duration on *in vivo* sensitivity of electromagnetic flow transducers. *Am. J. Physiol.* **236**, H508–H512.

Gross, R., Kirchheim, H., and Brandstetter, K. (1976). Basal vascular tone in the kidney: Evaluation from the static pressure-flow relationship under normal autoregulation and at maximum dilation in the dog. *Circ. Res.* **38**, 525–531.

Hohimer, A. R., and Smith, O. A. (1979). Decreased renal blood flow in the baboon during mild dynamic leg exercise. *Am. J. Physiol.* **236**, H141–H150.

Koch, E. (1931). "Die reflectorische Selbststeuerung des Kreislaufes." Steinkopff, Dresden.

Korner, P. I. (1971). Integrative neural cardiovascular control. *Physiol. Rev.* **51**, 312–367.

Rushmer, R. F. (1955). Applicability of Starling's law of the heart to intact unanesthetized animals. *Physiol. Rev.* **35**, 138–142.

Rushmer, R. F., and Smith, O. A. (1959). Cardiac control. *Physiol. Rev.* **39**, 41–68.

Smith, O. A., Hohimer, A. R., Astley, C., and Taylor, D. J. (1979). Renal and hindlimb vascular control during acute emotion in the baboon. *Am. J. Physiol.* **236**, R198–R205.

Smyth, H. S., Sleight, P., and Pickering, G. W. (1969). Reflex regulation of arterial pressure during sleep in man: A quantitative method of assessing baroreflex sensitivity. *Circ. Res.* **24**, 109–121.

Stephenson, R. B., and Smith, O. A. (1977). Behavior and vagal-sympathetic balance in the regulation of heart rate. *Fed. Proc., Fed. Am. Soc. Exp. Biol.* **36**, 441.

Stephenson, R. B., Smith, O. A., and Scher, A. M. (1975). Behavioral modulation of the baroreflex. *Physiologist* **18**, 408.

2

Brain Stem and
Cerebellar Mechanisms
of Cardiovascular Control

Jean C. Strahlendorf and Howard K. Strahlendorf

I. INTRODUCTION

Claude Bernard was the first to recognize the importance of the central nervous system (CNS) in the maintenance of homeostasis within the cardiovascular system when he made the observation that transection of the

NEURAL CONTROL OF CIRCULATION

cervical spinal cord caused a depressor response (Bernard, 1851). Later, in the mid to late 1800s, Owsjannikow and Dittmar (Owsjannikow, 1871; Dittmar, 1873) acknowledged that structures of the medulla oblongata may be sites involved in the control of cardiovascular dynamics. In the early 1900s, Bayliss (1901) introduced the concept of a bimodal vaso-motor center consisting of vasoconstrictor and vasodilator areas that acted reciprocally to govern vasomotor tone. Subsequently, direct bulbospinal effects on cardiovascular reflexes by stimulation of the floor of the fourth ventricle were reported in 1916 (Ranson and Billingsley, 1916), and were taken to represent evidence in favor of the postulated vasomotor areas of Bayliss. The classical studies of Alexander (1946) extended these ideas about the medullary cardiovascular centers by demonstrating that the caudal half of the medulla is a depressor center that is capable of toni-cally inhibiting the spinal cardiovascular center thereby reducing blood pressure, and that when the pressor center of the rostral medulla is ablated or removed, a similar decrease in both blood pressure and cardio-accelerator tone is seen. Current experimental evidence dictates that Bayliss's theory be modified to state that medullary control of vascular tone is effected almost entirely by variations in vasoconstrictor output and not via vasodilator activity. Medullary pressor and depressor areas have come to represent sites which affect vascular tone by excitation (or disinhibition) and inhibition, respectively, of spinal sympathetic vaso-constrictor neurons.

Since 1950 an extensive literature has developed concerning the func-tional organization of the brain stem and other CNS structures that may participate in the neural control of circulation (Smith, 1974; Calaresu et al., 1975; Wurster, 1977). The physiology and anatomy of medullary vasomotor reflexes initiated by the baroreceptors and chemo-receptors and subserved by baroceptive and chemoceptive fibers has re-ceived considerable attention (Korner, 1971; Sato, 1975). Furthermore, experimentally induced perturbations of these systems have become standard models for various cardiovascular pathologies, particularly hy-pertension. In the course of these investigations examining brain-stem medullary control of circulation, several new, interesting, and potentially important CNS structures have been discovered.

In the following sections, we will present a broad overview of the functional anatomy and physiology of the brain stem and cerebellar sites, which are becoming increasingly important in the understanding of central cardiovascular control. For a more thorough treatment of any one of these areas the reader should consult one of the other chapters con-tained in this volume or the review references cited.

II. THE BRAIN AS A GOVERNING FORCE IN CARDIOVASCULAR CONTROL

Much of the recent work that ascribes an important role to the central nervous system in the control of circulation is based on the premise that states that suprabulbar control mechanisms must interplay with barore-ceptors in order to obtain an increase in heart rate coincident with a rise in blood pressure (Bard, 1959). Although this insight has provided the necessary framework for today's research, credit also must be extended to Owsjannikow (1871) and Dittmar (1873), who located and described the vasomotor center in the mid-nineteenth century prior to the advent of the sphygmomanometer. These early research efforts helped to formulate the neurogenic concept for the central control of the cardiovascular system.

Julius (1976) has aptly summarized three major setbacks that may have been responsible for the skepticism underlying the importance of the neurogenic component of cardiovascular control. These include the less than spectacular results following surgical or chemical procedures employed to reduce sympathetic tone; the finding that blood vessels in a hypertensive person are hyperresponsive to vasoconstrictor influences; and the monumental observation that hypertension may be the consequence of the resetting of peripheral baroreceptor tone to a higher, less sensitive level, i.e., the baroreceptors cease to exhibit the usual responsiveness to elevated blood pressure.

In spite of these setbacks, the neurogenic concept gained favor following the advent of antihypertensive agents such as clonidine, various β-blockers, and α-methyldopa; drugs shown to act in the CNS, especially the brain stem, to effect a decrease in blood pressure. Studies designed to foster our comprehension and understanding of the neural control of the cardiovascular system will be instrumental for the future development of new drug therapies aimed at prevention or curtailment of cardiovascular pathologies. Sjoerdsma (1977) postulated that if there is one body organ whose function might be modified by a drug in such a way as to achieve a totally uncomplicated normalization of the blood pressure in hypertensive animals or man, this organ must be the brain.

III. FUNCTIONAL ANATOMY AND GENERAL ORGANIZATION OF THE LOWER BRAIN STEM

This section is designed as a cursory description of the general organization of the lower brain stem (Fig. 1), emphasizing areas relevant to

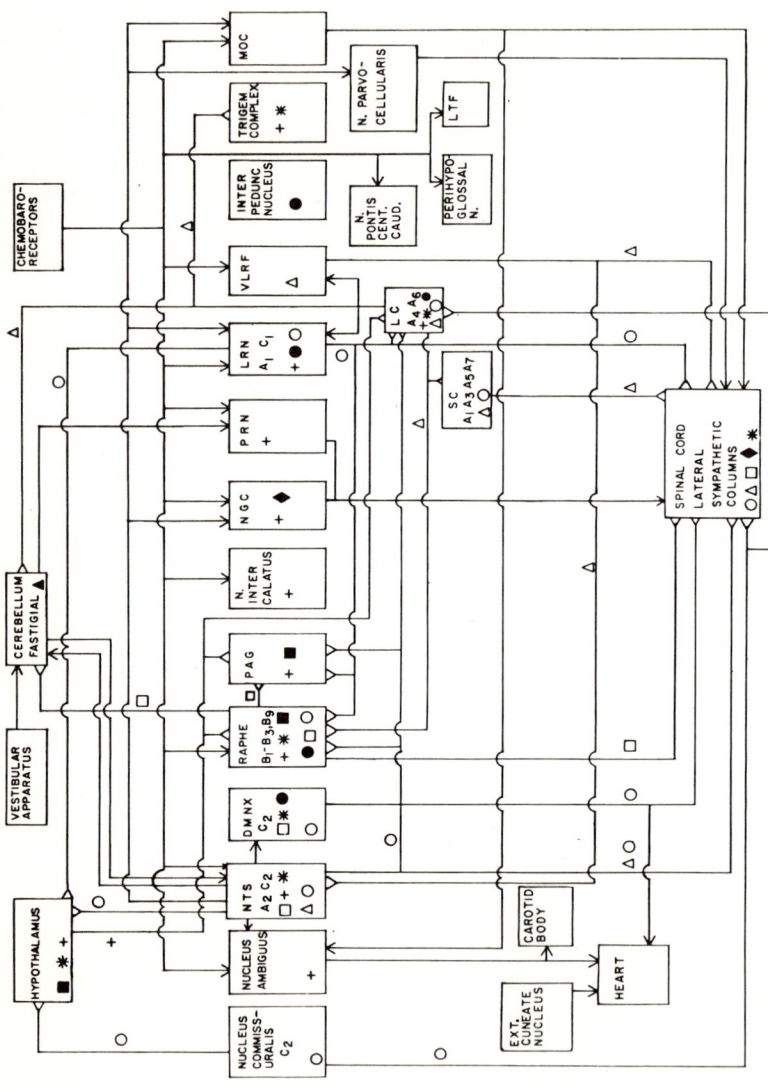

Fig. 1. The general organization of the lower brain stem. Abbreviations: DMNX, dorsal motor nucleus of vagus; INTERPEDUNC NUCLEUS, interpeduncular nucleus; LC, locus coeruleus; LRN, lateral reticular nucleus; LTF, lateral tegmental field; MOC, medulla oblongata centralis; NGC, nucleus gigantocellularis; N PONTIS CENT CAUD, nucleus pontis centralis caudalis; NTS, nucleus tractus solitarius; PAG, periaqueductal gray; PRN, paramedian reticular nucleus; SC, subcoeruleus; TRIGEM COMPLEX, trigeminal complex; VLRF, ventrolateral reticular formation. Substances: O, epinephrine; △, norepinephrine; □, 5-hydroxytryptamine; ●, acetylcholine; ▲, γ-aminobutyric acid; *, histamine; +, angiotensin; ■, endorphins and enkaphalins; ◆, substance P.

central control of the cardiovascular system. No attempt will be made to include speculative connections; only well-documented anatomical findings will be mentioned.

The concept of a medullary autonomic center, specifically the reticular formation, as a vasomotor center comprised of a highly specialized vasodepressor and vasoconstrictor component has been supplanted by a proposal that views the medulla as an integral part of a very complex integrative system originating from the cerebral cortex (Clarke *et al.*, 1968) and extending to the limbic system (Löfving, 1961), hypothalamus (Hilton and Spyer, 1971; Takeuchi and Manning, 1973), brain stem (Thomas and Calaresu, 1974), and the spinal cord (Pagani *et al.*, 1974). Studies have revealed that the medulla is not as highly compartmentalized as originally thought, and that activation of the classically defined vasodepressor and vasoconstrictor areas elicits mixed reactions on heart rate and blood pressure, due in part to the neuronal heterogenicity of the medullary reticular formation. It has been suggested that the medulla ultimately functions to integrate and maintain cardiovascular homeostasis (Reis, 1972).

A. Neural Input to the Lower Brain Stem

Baroreceptors and chemoreceptors relay circulatory information to the lower brain stem via the aortic depressor (aortic arch nerve, specifically the vagal branch) and the carotid sinus nerves (Cottle, 1964; Calaresu and Pearce, 1965; Humphrey, 1967; Crill and Reis, 1968; Kumada and Nakajima, 1972; Miura and Reis, 1972). The nucleus tractus solitarius, particularly that portion of the nucleus that lies near the obex (the intermediate third), is the main relay site in which afferent fibers of the carotid sinus nerve terminate; in turn, this nucleus projects to various brain stem areas. These sites, which are polysynaptically connected, include the raphé nuclei, lateral reticular nucleus, nucleus parvocellularis, and the nucleus pontis centralis caudalis. The paramedian reticular formation, nucleus medulla oblongata centralis, and nucleus gigantocellularis appear to receive direct and indirect cardiovascular input from baroreceptor and chemoreceptor afferents (Miura and Reis, 1969). Hellner and von Baumgarten (1961) speculated that the dorsal part of the nucleus tractus solitarius, an area whose cells fire in synchrony with the cardiac cycle, appear to receive vagal cardiovascular afferents. Anatomical evidence from studies in pigeons verifies a limited projection of vagal afferents to the dorsal nucleus tractus solitarius (Katz and Karten, 1979).

Employing intracellular techniques, Miura and Kitamura (1979) have recorded EPSPs of short latency (2–4 msec) and IPSPs of longer latency from the cells of nucleus tractus solitarius and the subjacent reticular formation. These findings provide evidence suggesting that the carotid sinus nerve exerts an inhibitory and excitatory influence on the nucleus tractus solitarius, and that other areas lying outside the boundary of the nucleus are monosynaptically excited by the carotid sinus nerve. The carotid sinus nerve-elicited EPSPs were generated within the nucleus ambiguus, lateral tegmental field, and perihypoglossal nucleus. Short and long latency IPSPs were observed within the dorsolateral quadrant of the paramedian reticular formation upon stimulation of the carotid sinus nerve. Therefore, in addition to the nucleus tractus solitarius, the paramedian reticular nucleus, nucleus ambiguus, lateral tegmental field and perihypoglossal nuclei receive direct monosynaptic excitatory and inhibitory input from the carotid sinus nerve.

B.   Neural Output from the Lower Brain Stem

Early studies in cats suggested that the dorsal motor nucleus of the vagus was the site of origin for the vagal cardioinhibitory fibers derived from within the medulla. However, electrical activation of this nucleus failed to produce negative chronotropic effects (Calaresu and Pearce, 1965). In addition, electrical stimulation of the peripheral vagus nerve in chronically prepared cats with lesioned dorsal motor nucleus of the vagus still produced bradycardia (Kerr, 1969). Laborde (1888) produced the first evidence that the nucleus ambiguus elicited bradycardia in the cat and dog following electrical activation. Numerous studies have addressed the issue as to which of these two nuclei is the site of origin of the vagal cardioinhibitory fibers. Basically, there appears to be a species-dependent difference in the distribution of these fibers. In cats, these fibers are located predominantly in the nucleus ambiguus (Sugimoto et al., 1979), although the dorsal motor nucleus of the vagus possesses some vagal soma; whereas, in pigeons, the cardioinhibitory neurons arise primarily from the dorsal motor nucleus of the vagus itself (Cohen and Schnall, 1970). Geis and Wurster (1978), utilizing subepicardiac injections of horseradish peroxidase in cats, revealed the presence of ipsilaterally labeled cell bodies within the nucleus ambiguus, dorsal motor nucleus of the vagus, and an intermediate zone between these two nuclear groups, with a preponderance of the soma (78%) located in the nucleus ambiguus. These investigators suggested that the cell bodies of the dorsal motor nucleus of the vagus control ventricular contractility, while nucleus ambiguus soma are involved in heart rate regulation. Consonant with these findings, Nosaka et al. (1979), employing horseradish peroxidase injections in rat hearts, saw reactive cells within the nucleus ambiguus, the dorsal motor nucleus of the vagus, and the intermediate area between these two nuclei.

Further implicating the region of the nucleus ambiguus as a site of origin of vagal efferent systems, DeGroat and co-workers (1979) have recently shown that this nucleus sends ipsilateral projections to the carotid body via the carotid sinus nerve. The nucleus ambiguus may give rise to the proposed efferent inhibitory pathway to the carotid body.

In addition to the nucleus ambiguus, Ciriello and Calaresu (1978) have proposed that the external cuneate nucleus may be a site of origin of cardioinhibitory axons, and probably functions as a component of reflex arcs which lead to cardiac slowing during arterial hypertension. Previous investigations had revealed terminal degeneration within the ventral portion of the external cuneate nucleus after sectioning the vagus and glossopharyngeal nerves (Sobusiak et al., 1972). Furthermore, electro-physiological data suggest that this nucleus has a monosynaptic connection with the aortic depressor nerve (Crill and Reis, 1968) as well as possessing individual units that fire synchronously with the heart beat (Middleton et al., 1965). Finally, lesions placed within the nucleus ambiguus did not alter the bradycardia/hypotension observed from electrical activation of the external cuneate nucleus, supportive of an independent role for this nucleus (Ciriello and Calaresu, 1978).

An extramedullary source of fibers to the cardiovascular effectors is the preganglionic neurons whose cell bodies lie in the vicinity of the intermediolateral spinal gray region of the spinal cord. The sympathetic preganglionic fibers which innervate the heart originate from C_8–T_1 to the L level of the spinal cord. The T_1–T_2 and L_3–L_4 segments are known to innervate the heart predominately (Wurster, 1977). In conjunction with the intermediolateral nucleus, sympathetic preganglionic cell bodies have been observed in the autonomic gray, the lateral funiculus, and the intercalated nucleus (Norris et al., 1974).

C. Central Interconnections within the Lower Brain Stem

This section presents findings concerning connections between input and output systems involved in cardiovascular reflexes within the medulla. Degenerative studies (Palkovits and Záborsky, 1977) involving lesions of the medial nucleus tractus solitarius resulted in axon and preterminal degeneration with the dorsal motor nucleus of vagus, in the nucleus intercalatus, and different subdivisions of the nucleus tractus solitarius. The presence of degenerative fibers within the nucleus tractus solitarius subsequent to the placement of small lesions in another part of the same nucleus exemplifies the complex intrinsic interconnections within this structure. Moderately dense degeneration was observed in the vicinity of nucleus ambiguus motoneurons with more diffuse degeneration within the nucleus reticularis lateralis, nucleus reticularis gigantocellularis, and nucleus reticularis medulla oblongata. Other investigators (Morest, 1967; Cottle and Calaresu, 1973) have traced degenerating fibers after nucleus tractus solitarius lesions to the ipsilateral nucleus ambiguus, the dorsal motor nucleus of the vagus, the retrofacial nucleus (rostral nucleus ambiguus), the dorsal tegmental nucleus, bilaterally to the ventrolateral portion of the nucleus intercalatus, and the nucleus prepositus hypoglossi.

The nucleus ambiguus, site of origin of vagal cardioinhibitory fibers, receives baroreceptor and chemoreceptor information from the nucleus tractus solitarius via the dorsal and ventral nucleus of the medulla oblongata centralis. Therefore, Thomas and Calaresu (1974) postulated that the nucleus ambiguus may complete the vagal pathway for baro- and chemoreceptor reflexes: vagal bradycardia resulted from electrical stimulation of the nucleus ambiguus, nucleus tractus solitarius, and the medulla oblongata centralis (Thomas and Calaresu, 1974).

In an attempt to identify the function of the medullary vasomotor centers, it has been shown electrophysiologically that nucleus parvocellularis, nucleus reticularis ventralis, the lateral reticular nucleus, and nucleus gigantocellularis exert an excitatory influence on the cardiovascular neurons of the spinal cord (Henry and Calaresu, 1974). The same cardiovascular spinal neurons were inhibited by the raphé nuclei, paramedian nucleus, and ventral nucleus medulla oblongata centralis (Henry and Calaresu, 1974). Kumada et al. (1979) have recently postulated that the "tonic vasomotor center" may be comprised of the parvocellular reticular nucleus, and the dorsal gigantocellularis (caudal part). This premise was partially based on the finding that lesions placed in these two areas elicited profound hypotension.

The caudal raphé nuclei (B_1, B_2, B_3) possess the majority of central serotonergic cell bodies whose axons descend into the spinal cord terminating in the sympathetic lateral column (Dahlström and Fuxe, 1965). Labeled protein and lesion studies revealed the presence of a direct projection from the rostral caudal extent of the medullary raphé to the cervical, thoracic, and lumbar spinal cord (Cabot et al., 1978). These authors also demonstrated an inhibitory influence of the medullary raphé on sympathetic preganglionic neurons. Electrical stimulation of the medullary raphé (B_1–B_3 groups) produced a depressor response with a concomitant decrease in systolic and diastolic pressure (Coote and MacLeod, 1974; Neumayr et al., 1974; Ward and Gunn, 1976), whereas selective chemical ablation of the bulbospinal serotonergic neurons produced an elevation of blood pressure (Ogawa, 1978). In contrast, electrical activation of the dorsal and median raphé nuclei elicited an increase in heart rate and blood pressure, possibly mediated by hypothalamic areas (Adair et al., 1977; Smits et al., 1978).

Much emphasis has been placed on the involvement of the locus coeruleus, a midbrain nucleus known to contain the highest concentration of norepinephrine in the central nervous system, on central control of blood pressure. Bilateral chemical destruction of the locus coeruleus by 6-hydroxydopamine in the Wistar-Kyoto (WKY) rat caused an elevation of both blood pressure and heart rate which lasted 2 weeks (Ogawa et al., 1977). Contrary to the lesion study, various investigators (Ward and Gunn, 1976; Kawamura et al., 1978) have elicited pressor responses to locus coeruleus stimulation, possibly the result of stimulation of an ascending fiber system to the posterior hypothalamus, and a descending fiber system to the ventral and lateral reticular formation (Ward and Gunn, 1976). Based on anatomical findings that describe posterior medial hypothalamic terminations within the locus coeruleus (Crosby and Woodburne, 1951; Mizuno and Nakamura, 1970) and the results of lesions of the locus coeruleus that abolished the pressor response after stimulation of the hypothalamus, Ward and Gunn (1976) speculated that the locus coeruleus-induced pressor response may be a component of the hypothalamic system.

Kawamura and his colleagues (1978) have recently observed in spontaneously hypertensive rats, certain response abnormalities following electrical activation of the locus coeruleus. Specifically, these animals displayed both a higher locus coeruleus pressor threshold than WKY control rats, and a depressor response not observed in the controls. The authors surmised that the pressor function of the locus coeruleus was simply less operative in the spontaneously hypertensive rats. The depressor response observed in the spontaneously hypertensive rats may reflect an increased sensitivity of their cardiovagal system. Therefore, the locus coeruleus may participate in the control of blood pressure in normotensive as well as hypertensive states.

The major descending pressor pathway of the spinal cord appears to be localized in the dorsolateral funiculus; maximal pressor responses are observed when an area approximately 2 mm ventrolateral to the dorsal lateral sulcus is stimulated. This pathway exerts a tonic regulatory influence on arterial pressure and is thought to be responsible for baroreceptor reflex alterations of blood pressure (Foreman and Wurster, 1973; Smirnov and Potekhina, 1974). Based on lesion studies, the right dorsolateral pathway exerts a more prominent influence on heart rate than does the left (Henry and Calaresu, 1972). Various investigators (Kuru *et al.*, 1960; Gebber *et al.*, 1973; Henry and Calaresu, 1974) have proposed that this pressor pathway may originate from the lateral-ventrolateral portion of the medullary reticular formation, which descends in the dorsolateral funiculus, terminating in the intermediolateral cell column.

Based on the premise that the sympathoexcitatory and vasopressor functions descend in the dorsolateral funiculus in cats (Foreman and Wurster, 1974) and rats (Schramm *et al.*, 1978, 1979b), Schramm *et al.* (1979a) performed bilateral lesions in the dorsolateral funiculus of spontaneously hypertensive rats to observe possible changes in the development of the genetic hypertension. Measurements of the intensity of the sympathetic silent period, an episode of profound sympathoinhibition or refractoriness which follows activation of central sympathetic pathways, was employed as an index of sympathetic excitability. These investigators found that lesions of the dorsolateral funiculus did not eliminate the relative sympathetic hyperexcitability observed in spontaneously hypertensive rats, nor prevent the development of hypertension.

IV. FUNCTIONAL ANATOMY AND GENERAL ORGANIZATION OF THE CEREBELLUM

Although experimentation concerning cerebellar function has emphasized somatomotor mechanisms, attention has recently focused on its involvement as an influential modulator of autonomic regulation (Hoffer, 1965; Reis and Cuénod, 1965; Smith and Nathan, 1966; Martner, 1975).

Phylogenetically, the cerebellum has been divided into three main regions: the archicerebellum, paleocerebellum, and neocerebellum. Newer texts subdivide the cerebellum according to a sagittal plane, the medial or vermis portion extending laterally as the intermediate or paravermis, which is bordered by the hemispheres. The medial area or vermis of the cerebellum and its projections to the fastigial nucleus appear to elicit the majority of autonomic responses. Anatomically, the cerebellar cortex is divided into three layers: the superficial or molecular layer that contains the inhibitory interneurons, i.e., superficial stellate and basket cells; the middle or ganglionic layer consisting of Purkinje cells; and the deep or granular layer that contains the excitatory granule cells and the Golgi cells, a type of inhibitory interneuron.

Purkinje cells receive two major types of facilitatory neuronal inputs: climbing fibers which end directly on Purkinje cells dendrites, and mossy fibers which excite granule cells whose axons traverse to the molecular layer and bifurcate to form the parallel fibers which then have endings on Purkinje cells. The ventral and dorsal spinocerebellar tracts (Miskolczy, 1931), external cuneate nucleus (Grant, 1962), lateral reticular nucleus and pontine nucleus (Snider, 1936) provide major mossy fiber input. The inferior olive appears to be the sole source of climbing fibers to the cerebellum (Szentágothai and Rajkovits, 1959). The Purkinje cell receives only one climbing fiber which terminates extensively upon the Purkinje cell dendrites. Mossy fibers produce through granular cells, a diffuse yet powerful direct excitation and an indirect inhibition of Purkinje cells; whereas, the climbing fiber input results in a direct monosynaptic excitation. The sole output of the cerebellar cortex is the Purkinje cell which inhibits the intracerebellar nuclear cell groups, i.e., fastigial nucleus, dentate nucleus, interpositus nucleus, and the lateral vestibular nucleus. For a more complete description of the cerebellum, readers are referred to the original work of Eccles *et al.* (1967).

V. CEREBELLAR INFLUENCES ON CENTRAL CARDIOVASCULAR CONTROL

Early investigations (Dresel and Lewy, 1924; Dow and Moruzzi, 1958) showed that electrical stimulation of the cerebellar cortex produced changes in heart rate and blood pressure; whereas, chronic cerebellar lesions failed to alter resting arterial pressure significantly. Subsequent studies demonstrated that cerebellar stimulation elicited a marked attenuation of vasomotor reflexes, without altering mean blood pressure (Moruzzi 1940; 1950). Specifically, vagal afferent activation and bilateral carotid occlusion, which normally elicited depressor and pressor responses, respectively, were inhibited on stimulation of the anterior lobe of the cerebellum. Accordingly, removal of the cerebellum enhanced vasomotor reflex activity in the decerebrate cat (Reis and Cuénod, 1965). Although the cerebellum does not appear to alter mean blood pressure significantly, it can markedly alter regional blood flow to the red skeletal muscle beds (Hoffer, 1965; Sheridan and Reis, 1972).

Recently, Kennedy (1978) hypothesized that the olivary nucleus in the medulla, the site of origin of climbing fiber input to the cerebellum, was involved in central control of blood pressure. Stimulation of the autonomic pathways from various diencephalic and midbrain structures that project to the medial portion of the olive caused a large sustained increase in blood pressure, although stimulation of the projectory site in the olive exerted no effect on blood pressure (Smith and Clarke, 1964). Furthermore, Smith and Nathan (1966) observed an indirect inhibitory influence of the olive on blood pressure; olive activation diminished the carotid sinus reflex in normotensive cats. Since the olive operates during motor learning (Gilbert and Thach, 1977), Kennedy (1978) postulated that this nucleus may affect blood pressure in certain circumstances, e.g., when motor tasks are being acquired or during exercise when an inhibitory influence on the carotid sinus reflex would maintain a hypertensive state.

It has been proposed that the cerebellum is involved in orthostatic control of blood pressure. In addition to baro-chemoreceptors, another source of peripheral receptors is the vestibular apparatus that registers changes in state when going from supine to a standing position and sends this information to the fastigial nucleus via the vestibular nerve (Doba and Reis, 1972). Electrical stimulation of the rostral medial fastigial nucleus causes a transient increase in heart rate and a rise in blood pressure, accompanied by vasoconstriction of arteries in limb, kidneys, and abdominal viscera (Achari and Downman, 1970; Lisander and Martner, 1971; Doba and Reis, 1972); these cardiovascular changes are also observed upon assumption of an upright position. Doba and Reis (1972) postulated that the fastigial nucleus is responsible for the increased sympathetic outflow initiated to compensate for orthostatic hypotension. In this light, bilateral lesions of the fastigial nucleus impaired reflex cardiovascular responses to tilting (Doba and Reis, 1972). Lisander and Martner (1971) correlated the cardiovascular responses elicited after fastigial nucleus stimulation to that of baroreceptor unloading. For example, fastigial activation suppressed bradycardia normally elicited by norepinephrine and phenylbiguanide injections (Achari *et al.*, 1973) and afferent sinus and vagus nerve stimulation (Hockman *et al.*, 1970).

Since the paramedian reticular formation receives inputs from both the baroreceptor/chemoreceptor afferents and the fastigial nucleus, Miura and Reis (1971) proposed that it may mediate the influence of the fastigial nucleus on orthostatic hypotension. Furthermore, bilateral lesions of the paramedian reticular nucleus were shown to reduce the fastigial-elicited pressor response (Doba and Reis, 1972).

Fastigial mediated hypertension appears to be due to activation of sympathoexcitatory paths coursing bilaterally within the dorsolateral column of the spinal cord. Moreover, the cardiovascular effects observed on activation of the fastigial nucleus may relate to the anatomical findings that revealed that reciprocal connections exist between the fastigial nucleus and the parasolitary portion of the nucleus tractus solitarius (Batton *et al.*, 1977) as well as the nucleus paramedian reticularis, both implicated in baroreceptor activity.

Recently, Hennemann and Rubia (1978) recorded field potentials on the cerebellar cortex in response to cervical vagus stimulation; maximum amplitudes were recorded in a bilateral sagittal strip across lobules V and VI and on the paramedian lobule. On the basis of this distribution and the field potential profiles, it was suggested that the potentials had their origin in the inferior olive and were carried to the cerebellar cortex via the climbing fiber system. Interestingly, the location of the area of maximum activity corresponded to the sagittal projection of the lateral funiculus spino-olivo-cerebellar pathway (Larson *et al.*, 1969; Armstrong *et al.*, 1973). This study represents an important electrophysiologic demonstration of autonomic input to the cerebellum.

VI. NEUROTRANSMITTERS POTENTIALLY INVOLVED IN CENTRAL CARDIOVASCULAR REGULATION

A. Acetylcholine

Involvement of CNS cholinergic processes in regulatory mechanisms important to central control of cardiovascular dynamics is poorly understood. This derives in part from a lack of adequate localization and mapping of acetylcholine containing neurons in the brain. With regard to structures presumed important to central autonomic regulation, acetylcholine has been localized in relatively high concentrations in the nuclei of the cranial nerves including dorsal motor nucleus of the vagus, in the dorsal raphé complex, and interpeduncular nucleus (McGeer *et al.*, 1978). Moderate to high concentrations of acetylcholine are also present in the locus coeruleus and the lateral reticular formation (Cheney *et al.*, 1975).

The influence of central cholinergic neurotransmission on blood pressure regulation has been extensively studied using pharmacologic interventions injected directly into brain sites or into the ventricular cavities. The lateral medullary reticular formation contains numerous cholinoceptive sites which can affect blood pressure. Activation of nicotinic receptors in this area generally elicits a systemic pressor response; whereas, muscarinic agents usually lower blood pressure when applied to this reticular area via microinjection. Acetylcholine applied to the floor of fourth ventricle, however, has been shown to evoke only a pressor action (Tangri *et al.*, 1977). Day and Roach (1977) have speculated that these centrally induced pressor effects are mediated via increased sympathetic outflow since they can be abolished by peripheral adrenergic blockade. The cholinergic agonist carbachol when injected into the fourth ventricle or dorsal medulla just rostral to the nucleus tractus solitarius elicits a biphasic response consisting of a transient depressor action followed by prolonged hypertension. Mecamylamine or hexamethonium effectively attenuated carbachol actions, indicating a nicotinic receptor mechanism (Brezenoff and Jenden, 1970). Finally, it has been proposed that intraventricular carbachol elicits its blood pressure effects indirectly via an interaction between cholinergic and noradrenergic or adrenergic systems, since prior intraventricular administration of propranolol or guanethidine abolishes the cardiovascular actions of the cholinergic agonist (Day and Roach, 1977).

A clearer understanding of the role of the central cholinergic system awaits further elucidation of both neuronal networks utilizing this compound as a neurotransmitter and of central structures which govern or modulate the autonomic system.

B.   Serotonin

Serotonin-containing cell bodies are localized almost exclusively in the raphé complex. Descending serotonin neurons arise mainly from areas termed B_1 and B_2, the midline raphé nuclei, and from B_3, an area slightly more lateral in the brain stem (Dahlström and Fuxe, 1965). These fibers course in the lateral funiculi of the spinal cord and terminate in gray matter of the horns with a particularly dense innervation to the sympathetic intermediolateral cell column (Fuxe et al., 1968). Neurons from raphé extend rostrally to innervate the pontine reticular formation, periaqueductal gray, and the Fields of Forel of the posterior hypothalamus and extend dorsally into the cerebellum where anatomical studies have revealed atypical nonsynaptic terminations suggestive of a neurohumoral modulatory function (Chan-Palay, 1977). The highest levels of serotonin outside the raphé proper occur in the basal and posterior hypothalamus (Saavedra et al., 1974). The dorsal and more rostral raphé nuclei receive a dense innervation from the locus coeruleus (Antonaccio, 1977), and some reports have demonstrated a projection from the raphé back to the locus coeruleus (Descarries and Leger, 1978). These anatomical findings have been supported by electrophysiological studies (Strahlendorf et al., 1979).

Electrical stimulation of the raphé nuclei causes a fall in blood pressure and decreased sympathetic outflow via the bulbospinal pathway that terminates on spinal preganglionic sympathoexcitatory neurons (Neumayr et al., 1974). Ascending and lateral inhibition occurs in the midbrain and pontine reticular formation (Nakamura, 1975). Pharmacologic activation of central serotonin receptors generally causes hypotension and bradycardia, possibly as a result of a decrease in overall sympathetic outflow over the cardiac, splanchnic, and renal nerves (Baum and

Shropshire, 1975). Serotonergic systems therefore appear to exert a generalized inhibition of sympathetic activity at several levels of the neuroaxis.

C. Epinephrine

Epinephrine-containing cell bodies are found in the nucleus reticularis lateralis (C_1) of the medulla oblongata (Hökfelt *et al.,* 1974) and in a complex of cell groups in or near the nucleus tractus solitarius, vagal nuclei, and nucleus commissuralis (C_2) near the A_2 group of the norepinephrine system described by Dahlström and Fuxe (1965). Collectively these areas project to restricted areas of the brain stem and spinal cord. Epinephrine-containing terminals are found in the sympathetic lateral columns, dorsal vagal motor nucleus, and nucleus tractus solitarius as well as hypothalamic and other periventricular structures. There is also substantial innervation of the locus coeruleus and raphé nuclei (Hökfelt *et al.,* 1974). As such this system is anatomically well suited to participate in central control of cardiovascular functions.

On the basis of recent experimental findings, it has been proposed that epinephrine-containing neurons may represent a central depressor system, while norepinephrine neurons may represent a central pressor system (Fuxe *et al.,* 1975). Structures such as the hypothalamus, nucleus tractus solitarius, dorsal motor nucleus of the vagus and the lateral columns receive rich dual innervation, i.e., epinephrine and norepinephrine. Thus, the balance between central epinephrine and norepinephrine receptor activity can conceivably play a crucial role in blood pressure homeostasis.

D. Norepinephrine

The norepinephrine-containing neurons of the midbrain and brain stem comprise the most heavily investigated neurotransmitter system with respect to central blood pressure control. Highest concentrations of norepinephrine-containing neurons are localized in the locus coeruleus (A_6) and subcoeruleus (A_7). In addition to dense interconnections between these two areas, a system of ascending and descending noradrenergic neurons arises from these nuclei. Axons from the locus coeruleus innervate the cerebellum, superior and inferior colliculi, spinal trigeminal nucleus, upper brain stem, medullary reticular formation, basal forebrain, cerebral cortex, and the hypothalamus (Dahlström and Fuxe, 1965). There is dense noradrenergic innervation of the dorsal motor nucleus of the vagus and nucleus tractus solitarius (Dahlström and Fuxe,

1965). Within the nucleus tractus solitarius, catecholamine receptor sites are located in the mediocaudal part (A_2 region) (Zanberg and De Jong, 1977) with norepinephrine-containing terminals originating from the A_1 and A_2 catecholamine cell groups (Wijnen et al., 1978). The A_1 and A_2 regions together with the nucleus commissuralis receive direct input from peripheral vascular receptors (Wijnen et al., 1978). Descending noradrenergic tracts arise from cells in the ventrolateral reticular formation (A_1), the subcoeruleus complex, and from area A_2, corresponding to the nucleus tractus solitarius and vagal complex (Dahlström and Fuxe, 1965). Axons from these areas course in the lateral funiculi and terminate in the dorsal and ventral horns as well as the intermediolateral cell columns (Antonaccio, 1977).

Studies examining the influence of central noradrenergic pathways on cardiovascular function have yielded a myriad of results. Generally, three central norepinephrine-containing neuron systems may contribute to the control of blood pressure (Starke et al., 1976). The central part of the baroreflex arc appears to be influenced by noradrenergic neurons, perhaps those innervating the nucleus tractus solitarius: stimulation of this pathway is believed to enhance the baroreceptor depressor reflex and hence lower blood pressure. Second, activation of ascending noradrenergic pathways from the locus coeruleus elicits increases in blood pressure. In comparison, clonidine, a centrally active hypotensive agent, exerts profound inhibition on coerulear cells when applied microiontophoretically (Aghajanian, 1978). Third, activation of descending bulbospinal noradrenergic pathways, possibly those terminating in the intermediolateral cell groups, appears to increase blood pressure. Given the inherent anatomical and physiological complexities of these systems a great deal more work is necessary before a comprehensive picture of catecholamines in central cardiovascular control can be drawn.

E. Amino Acids

Of the many putative neurotransmitters, glycine, γ-amino butyric acid (GABA), taurine, glutamate and aspartate are probably the best accepted candidates for amino acid mediated neurotransmission. Regional distribution and mapping of neurons containing any of these compounds is still in the embryonic stage, and as a consequence, their respective roles as mediators or modulators of central cardiovascular control are, at best, primitive and speculative.

Glycine, GABA, and taurine are generally regarded as inhibitory neurotransmitters, i.e., when applied to neural elements they suppress cell firing. In the monkey, high concentrations of GABA have been demonstrated in deep cerebellar nuclei including the fastigial nucleus (Fahn and Cote, 1968), a nucleus which is known to produce a strong pressor response when chemically (glutamate) or electrically activated (Dormer *et al.,* 1977). Glycine is present in high concentrations in the pons and medulla, but the exact location and pattern of distribution is unclear. Glycine may act as a transmitter in some descending inhibitory bulbospinal pathways and as the transmitter mediating commissural inhibition of vestibular neurons (Precht *et al.,* 1973) whose function may be involved with the cerebellum in regard to orthostatic cardiovascular control. Introduction of glycine or GABA into the third ventricle of cats has been shown to elicit depressor responses with bradycardia and decreased renal nerve discharge. These responses were thought to arise via a reduction in vasomotor tone from the caudal medulla (Guertzenstein, 1973; Antonaccio and Taylor, 1977). A recent report indicates that GABA-nergic synapses may comprise part of the reflex vagal pathway (Gillis and Williford, 1979), and GABA agonists such as muscimol appear to decrease blood pressure and heart rate by an action on the anterior medulla (Snyder *et al.,* 1979). Although taurine concentration is high in the pons, there is no evidence to date to suggest that taurine plays a regulatory role in central blood pressure control (Nara *et al.,* 1978).

Excitant amino acids such as glutamate and aspartate accelerate cell firing in a nonspecific manner by an action on the soma. Because studies examining the regional distribution of these amino acids are lacking and owing to the nonspecific nature of excitation by these compounds, little can be said presently regarding their function in the neural regulation of the cardiovascular system. Generally, injection of these substances into proposed central regulative sites mimics the cardiovascular effects of electrical stimulation.

F. Histamine

Histamine is present in the central nervous system of mammals in two pools: extraneuronal (mast cells) and neuronal; histamine in the latter locale has been proposed as a neurotransmitter. It is synthesized by a specific decarboxylase localized in the cytoplasm of nerve endings, partly stored in synaptic vesicles, and depolarization causes its release and accelerates its synthesis (Brown *et al.,* 1959). Enzymes responsible for its catabolism are also present (Schwartz, 1975). Recently, evidence accrued from lesion studies has suggested the presence of a network of histamine-containing neurons within the brain, ascending from the brain stem and coursing rostrally though the lateral hypothalamus via the medial forebrain bundle (Garbarg *et al.*, 1973; 1974). There is little or no evidence indicating a descending projection or defining collaterals of the ascending system into the caudal medulla and brain stem. Large regional differences in histamine levels have been reported in the rat (Taylor and Snyder, 1971), monkey (Taylor *et al.*, 1972), and man (Lipinski *et al.*, 1973), although caution must be exercised in interpreting these results since as much as 50% of brain histamine is contained in nonneuronal elements (Schwartz, 1977). Highest histamine levels are present in the hypothalamus, particularly the supraoptic nucleus and mammillary bodies while lowest levels are found in the cerebellum and pontine medullary regions (Calcutt, 1976).

Histamine as a mediator or modulator of central cardiovascular function has received relatively little attention, perhaps due to the paucity of identified histaminergic neurons in brain stem cardiovascular sites. In this regard, histamine is found in highest concentrations in the central gray and raphé nuclei (McGeer *et al.*, 1978). Intraventricularly administered histamine in cats and rats elicits short-lived increases in blood pressure with tachycardia, which may reflect an increased sympathetic tone (Finch and Hicks, 1976). In dogs, histamine is active at the level of the area postrema to produce emesis as a result of chemoreceptor trigger zone stimulation (Bhargava and Dixit, 1968). Microiontophoretic application of histamine to single neurons of cat medulla and brain stem elicited predominantly depressant actions (Haas *et al.*, 1973). The lack of an identified histaminergic input to the cells tested precludes a meaningful interpretation of these results.

G. Neuropeptides

1. *Angiotensin*

All components of an isorenin–angiotensin system, including angiotensinogen, isorenin, angiotensin I, angiotensin I-converting enzymes, angiotensin II, angiotensin receptors, and angiotensinases are present in brain (Ganten *et al.*, 1977). Immunofluorescence studies have revealed a regional distribution of angiotensin in the CNS (Fuxe *et al.*, 1976). Areas with particularly high density include the substantia gelatinosa of the spinal cord, spinal nucleus of the trigeminal nerve, median eminence, central amygdaloid nucleus, and the sympathetic lateral columns. The locus coeruleus appears to have a moderate concentration of angiotensin while scattered terminals are found in the periventricular gray of the pons and medulla, hypothalamus, reticular formation, raphé nuclei, nucleus tractus solitarius, and dorsal vagal motor nucleus, as well as other forebrain and limbic structures. It has also been shown that isorenin and angiotensin II are located intracellularly in nerve endings (Fuxe *et al.,* 1976), and there is considerable overlap in the distribution of angiotensin and norepinephrine in brain (Fisher-Ferraro *et al.,* 1971). Isorenin activity is known to be present in synaptosome fractions of brain homogenates that also contain catecholamines.

Central administration of angiotensin either intraventricularly or intracisternally elicits a marked increase in systemic blood pressure, an effect thought to arise from a direct action on the area postrema of the medulla (Ferrario *et al.,* 1972). Of particular interest in this regard is the fact that the area postrema lacks a blood–brain barrier thereby exposing it to additional actions of systemically circulating peptide. It has been postulated (Antonaccio, 1977) that the central pressor actions could result from disinhibition of descending facilitatory monoaminergic tracts as a consequence of decreasing inhibitory drives arising in the bulbar reticular formation. In this respect the area postrema lies in particularly close proximity to the nucleus tractus solitarius-vagal complex. Other sites important for the full expression of central angiotensin activity include the hypothalamus, midbrain, (Gildenberg, 1969) and the subnucleus medialis of the periaqueductal gray (Buckley, 1977). Angiotensin inhibits the reuptake of norepinephrine released by nerve impulses and taken collectively with data indicating a close regional association of these compounds, it would appear that perhaps angiotensin acts to modulate central noradrenergic neurotransmission in areas that participate in cardiovascular control.

2. Endorphins and Enkephalins

Since the discovery and characterization of the various endogenous opiate peptides, an extensive amount of work has been devoted to mapping and defining the regional distribution of the endorphins and enkephalins. In general, the endorphins are contained in a network of long axons radiating outward rostrally and caudally from an area within, and dorsolateral to, the hypothalamic arcuate nucleus. Midbrain and brain stem areas which receive the heaviest innervation include the noradrenergic cells of the locus coeruleus, the raphé nuclei (particularly the dorsal component), and the mesencephalic periaqueductal gray (Bloom *et al.,* 1978). In contrast to the long axon endorphin system, enkephalins are usually localized in short axon internuncial cells throughout the central nervous system. Such distribution and connections suggest neuroregulatory or neuromodulatory roles for these compounds. Within the pons, numerous nerve terminals are located in the dorsal parabrachial nucleus, locus coeruleus, and periaqueductal central gray (Johansson *et al.,* 1978). More caudally in the medulla, enkephalin terminals are found in the nucleus ambiguus, nucleus tractus solitarius, lateral reticular nucleus, nucleus intercalatus, and the nuclei of the facial, hypoglossal, and trigeminal nerves. The distribution of opiate receptors in the lower medulla has been examined and corresponds closely with those areas demonstrating enkephalin nerve terminals; these represent potentially important structures for cardiovascular control. In addition to the above-mentioned terminal areas, enkephalin-containing nerve cell bodies are found in the interpeduncular nucleus, lateral lemniscus, ventral and dorsal parabrachial nucleus, medial vestibular nucleus, nuclei raphé magnus and pallidus, ventromedial aspect of the nucleus gigantocellularis, nucleus tractus solitarius, and the paramedian reticular nucleus (Johansson *et al.,* 1978). Many of these structures have important implications with regard to the central neural regulation of circulation.

Several studies have investigated the central effects of opiates on cardiovascular responses. Morphinomimetics have been shown to facilitate baroreceptor reflexes at the level of the nucleus tractus solitarius, and to induce vagal-mediated bradycardia with a concomitant decrease in sympathetic tone—actions hypothesized to arise in part from the nucleus ambiguus (Laubie *et al.,* 1977; Daskalopoulos *et al.,* 1975). Met-enkephalin applied to the ventral surface of the brain stem produced a biphasic response consisting of an initial short duration pressor response followed by a longer duration and larger magnitude decline in blood pressure (Flórez and Mediavilla, 1977). Cells of the lateral reticular nucleus are inhibited by opiates and opiate peptides, while neurons of the nucleus gigantocellularis and paragigantocellularis exhibit either depression or excitation to morphinomimetics (Spring and Haigler, 1979; Satoh *et al.,* 1979). More rostrally, the nucleus locus coeruleus is extremely sensitive to the depressant actions of morphine and endogenous opiate peptides and is also markedly inhibited by clonidine, a centrally acting hypotensive agent (Aghajanian, 1978; Strahlendorf *et al.,* 1980).

Given the marked similarities between anatomical structures thought to play a role in the central regulation of autonomic function (particularly those rich in catecholamines) and the regional distribution of endogenous opiates and opiate receptors, it is likely that these peptides function in some regulatory manner within these areas. The exact nature of this interplay is a subject which deserves a great deal more study.

VII. SUMMARY

Significant anatomical advances have been made regarding central regions involved in the control of the cardiovascular system. Furthermore, the neurochemistry of these regions is becoming available with the advent of new sensitive techniques. Obviously, a large gap exists between the knowledge currently held and a full understanding of how the brain orchestrates the autonomic nervous system. A close and continued analysis of the physiology and synaptology of the interconnections of these areas seems warranted. Furthermore, more emphasis should be placed on the role of the new peptides, such as the endorphins, as well as some of the less investigated amines and amino acids. In light of the recent evidence demonstrating direct interactions between various neurotransmitter systems, further studies should be designed to consider these possible interrelationships in formulating a more comprehensive description of central autonomic control.

This overview has primarily focused on the regulative and coordinative functions of the brain stem and cerebellum on central blood pressure control. These areas are only part of a more extensive system. The physiological hierarchy of the central nervous system, in addition to various psychological factors which contribute to cardiovascular pathologies, necessitate an integrative theory which includes functions of the cerebral cortex and the limbic system.

REFERENCES

Achari, N. K., and Downman, C. B. B. (1970). Autonomic effector responses to stimulation of nucleus fastigius. *J. Physiol. (London)* **210,** 637–650.

Achari, N. K., Al-Ubaidy, S., and Downman, C. B. B. (1973). Cardiovascular responses elicited by fastigial and hypothalamic stimulation in conscious cats. *Brain Res.* **60,** 439–447.

Adair, J. R., Hamilton, B. L., Scappaticci, K. A., Helke, C. J., and Gillis, R. A. (1977). Cardiovascular responses to electrical stimulation of the medullary raphé area of the cat. *Brain Res.* **128,** 141–145.

Aghajanian, G. K. (1978). Tolerance of locus coeruleus neurones to morphine and suppression of withdrawal response by clonidine. *Nature (London)* **276,** 186–188.

Alexander, R. S. (1946). Tonic and reflex functions of medullary sympathetic cardiovascular centers. *J. Neurophysiol.* **9,** 205–217.

Antonaccio, M. J. (1977). Neuropharmacology of central mechanisms governing the circulation. *In* "Cardiovascular Pharmacology" (M. Antonaccio, ed.), p. 143. Raven, New York.

Antonaccio, M. J., and Taylor, D. G. (1977). Involvement of central GABA receptors in the regulation of blood pressure and heart rate of anesthetized cats. *Eur. J. Pharmacol.* **46,** 283–287.

Armstrong, D. M., Harvey, R. J., and Schild, R. F. (1973). Spino-olivo-cerebellar pathways to the posterior lobe of the cat cerebellum. *Exp. Brain Res.* **18,** 1–18.

Bard, P. (1959). Anatomical organization of the central nervous system in relation to control of the heart and blood vessels. *Physiol. Res.* **40** Suppl. 4, 3–26.

Batton, R. R., III, Jayaraman, A., Ruggiero, D., and Carpenter, M. B. (1977). Fastigial efferent projections in the monkey: An autoradiographic study. *J. Comp. Neurol.* **174,** 281–306.

Baum, T., and Shropshire, A. T. (1975). Inhibition of efferent sympathetic nerve activity by 5-hydroxytryptophan and centrally-administered 5-hydroxytryptamine. *Neuropharmacology* **14**, 227–233.

Bayliss, W. M. (1901). On the origin from the spinal cord of the vasodilator fibers of the hindlimb, and on the nature of these fibers. *J. Physiol.* **26**, 173.

Bernard, C. M. (1851). Influence du grand sympathique sur la sensibilité et sur la calorification. *C. R. Soc. Biol.* **3**, 163–164.

Bhargava, K. P., and Dixit, K. S. (1968). Role of the chemoreceptor trigger zone in histamine-induced emesis. *Br. J. Pharmacol.* **34**, 508–513.

Bloom, F. E., Rossier, J., Battenberg, E. L. F., Bayon, A., French, E., Henriksen, S. J., Siggins, G. R., Segal, D., Browne, R., Ling, R., and Guillemin, R. (1978). β-Endorphin: Cellular localization, electrophysiological and behavioral effects. *In* Advances in Biochemical Psychopharmacology, Vol. 18" (E. Costa and M. Trabucchi, eds.), pp. 89–109. Raven Press, New York.

Brezenoff, H. E., and Jenden, D. J. (1970). Changes in arterial blood pressure after micro-injection of carbachol into the medulla and IV ventricle of rat brain. *Neuropharmacology* **9**, 341–348.

Brown, D. D., Tomchick, R., and Axelrod, J. (1959). The distribution and properties of a histamine-methylating enzyme. *J. Biol. Chem.* **234**, 2948–2950.

Buckley, J. P. (1977). Central vasopressor actions of angiotensin. *Biochem. Pharmacol.* **26**, 1–3.

Cabot, J. B., Wild, J. M., and Cohen, D. H. (1978). Anatomical, physiological and behavioral evidence for medullary raphé inhibition of sympathetic preganglionic neurons. *Soc. Neurosci. Abstr.* **4**, 17.

Calaresu, F. R., and Pearce, J. W. (1965). Effects on heart rate of electrical stimulation of medullary vagal structures in the cat. *J. Physiol. (London)* **176**, 241–251.

Calaresu, F. R., Faiers, A. A., and Mogenson, G. J. (1975). Central neural regulation of heart and blood vessels in mammals. *Prog. Neurobiol. (Oxford)* **5**, 3–35.

Calcutt, C. R. (1976). Minireview: The role of histamine in the brain. *Gen. Pharmacol.* **7**, 15–25.

Chan-Palay, V. (1977). The indoleamine afferent axons to the cerebellum. *In* "Cerebellar Dentate Nucleus: Organization, Cytology, and Transmitters," pp. 390–454. Springer-Verlag, Berlin and New York.

Cheney, D. L., LaFevre, H. F., and Racagni G. (1975). Choline acetyltransferase activity and mass fragmentographic measurement of actylcholine in specific nuclei and tracts of rat brain. *Neuropharmacology* **14**, 801–809.

Ciriello, J., and Calaresu, F. R. (1978). Vagal bradycardia elicited by stimulation of the external cuneate nucleus in the cat, *Am. J. Physiol.* **235**, R286–R293.

Clarke, N. P., Smith, O. A., and Shearn, D. W. (1968). Topographical representation of limbs in primate motor cortex. *Am. J. Physiol.* **214**, 122–129.

Cohen, D. H., and Schnall, A. M. (1970). Medullary cells of origin of vagal cardioinhibitory fibers in the pigeon. II. Electrical stimulation of the dorsal motor nucleus. *J. Comp. Neurol.* **140**, 299–320.

Coote, J. H., and MacLeod, V. H. (1974). The influence of bulbospinal monoaminergic pathways on sympathetic nerve activity. *J. Physiol. (London)* **241**, 453–475.

Cottle, M. K. (1964). Degeneration studies of primary afferents of IXth and Xth cranial nerves in the cat. *J. Comp. Neurol.* **122**, 329–345.

Cottle, M. K. W., and Calaresu, F. R. (1973). Some terminal regions of secondary visceral afferents. *Can. Physiol.* **4**, 173.

Crill, W. E., and Reis, D. J. (1968). Distribution of carotid sinus and depressor nerves in cat brain stem. *Am. J. Physiol.* **214**, 269–276.

Crosby, E. C., and Woodburne, R. T. (1951). The mammalian midbrain and isthmus regions. Part II, The fiber connections. C. The hypothalamotegmental pathways. *J. Comp. Neurol.* **94,** 1–32.

Dahlström, A., and Fuxe, K. (1965). Evidence of the existence of monamine neurons in the central nervous system. I. Demonstration of monoamines in the cell bodies of neurons. IV. Distribution of monoamine nerve terminals in the central nervous system. *Acta Physiol. Scand. Suppl.* **247,** 37–84.

Daskalopoulous, N. Th., Laubie, M., and Schmitt, H. (1975). Localization of the central sympatho-inhibitory effect of a narcotic analgesic agent, fentanyl, in cats. *Eur. J. Pharmacol.* **33,** 91–97.

Day, M. D., and Roach, A. G. (1977). Cardiovascular effects of carbachol and other cholinomimetics administered into the cerebral ventricles of conscious cats. *Clin. Exp. Pharmacol. Physiol.* **4,** 431–442.

DeGroat, W. C., Nadelhaft, I., Morgan, C., and Schauble, T. (1979). The central origin of efferent pathways in the carotid sinus nerve of the cat. *Science* **205,** 1017–1018.

Descarries, L., and Leger, L. (1978). Serotonin nerve terminals in the locus coeruleus of the adult rat. *In* "Interactions between Putative Neurotransmitters in the Brain" (S. Garattini, J. F. Pujol and R. Samanin, eds.), pp. 355–367. Raven, New York.

Dittmar, C. (1873). Uber die lage des sogenannten gefasscentrums der medulla oblongata. *Ber. Verh. Sächs Akad. Wiss. Leipzig Math.-Phys. Kl.* **25,** 449–479.

Doba, N., and Reis, D. J. (1972). Cerebellum: role in reflex cardiovascular adjustment to posture. *Brain Res.* **39,** 495–500.

Dormer, K. R., Foreman, R. D., and Stone, H. L. (1977). Glutamate-induced fastigial pressor response in the dog. *Neuroscience* **2,** 577–584.

Dow, R. S., and Moruzzi, G. (1958). "The Physiology and Pathology of the Cerebellum." Univ. of Minnesota Press, Minneapolis, Minnesota.

Dresel, K., and Lewy, F. H. (1924). Die lokalisation vegetativer zentren im kleinhirn. *Dtsch. Z. Nervenheilkd.* **81,** 82–83.

Eccles, J. C., Ito, M., and Szentagothai, J. (1967). *In* "The Cerebellum as a Neuronal Machine." Springer-Verlag, Berlin and New York.

Fahn, S., and Cote, L. (1968). Regional distribution of γ-aminobutyric acid (GABA) in brain of rhesus monkey. *J. Neurochem.* **15,** 209–213.

Ferrario, C. M., Gildenberg, P. L., and McCubbin, J. W. (1972). Cardiovascular effects of angio-tensin mediated by the central nervous system. *Circ. Res.* **30,** 257–262.

Finch, L., and Hicks, P. E. (1976). Central hypertensive action of histamine in concious normotensive cats. *Eur. J. Pharmacol.* **36,** 263–266.

Fisher-Ferraro, C., Nahmod, V. E., Goldstein, D. J., and Finkielman, S. (1971). Angiotensin and renin in rat and dog brain. *J. Exp. Med.* **133,** 353–361.

Flórez, J., and Mediavilla, A. (1977). Respiratory and cardiovascular effects of met-enkephalin applied to the ventral surface of the brain stem. *Brain Res.* **138,** 585–590.

Foreman, R. D., and Wurster, R. D. (1973). Localization and functional characteristics of descending sympathetic spinal pathways. *Am. J. Physiol.* **225,** 212–217.

Foreman, R. D., and Wurster, R. D. (1974). Conduction on descending spinal pathways initiated by somato-sympathetic reflexes. *Am. J. Physiol.* **228,** 905–908.

Fuxe, K., Hökfelt, T., and Ungerstedt, U. (1968). Localisation of indolealkylamines in CNS. *Adv. Pharmacol.* **6A,** 235–251.

Fuxe, K., Hökfelt, T., Bolme, P., Goldstein, M., Johansson, O., Jonsson, G., Lidbrink, P., Ljungdahl, A., and Sachs, Ch. (1975). The topography of central catecholamine pathways in relation to their possible role in blood pressure control. *In* "Central

Action of Drugs in Blood Pressure Regulation" (D. S. Davies and J. L. Reid, eds.), pp. 8–23. Univ. Park Press, Baltimore, Maryland.

Fuxe, K., Ganten, D., Hökfelt, T., and Bolme, P. (1976). Immunohistochemical evidence for the existence of angiotensin II-containing nerve terminals in the brain and spinal cord of the rat. *Neurosci. Lett.* **2**, 229–234.

Ganten, D., Fuxe, K., Ganten, U., Hökfelt, T., and Bolme, P. (1977). The brain isorenin-angiotensin system: Localization and biological function. *In* "Progress in Brain Research, Vol. 47, Hypertension and Brain Mechanisms" (W. De Jong, A. P. Provoost and A. P. Shapiro, eds.), pp. 155–165. Elsevier, Amsterdam.

Garbarg, M., Krishnamoorthy, M. S., Feger, J., and Schwartz, J. C. (1973). Effects of mesencephalic and hypothalamic lesions on histamine levels in rat brain. *Brain Res.* **50**, 361–367.

Garbarg, M., Barbin, G., Feger, J., and Schwartz, J. C. (1974). Histaminergic pathways in rat brain evidenced by lesions of the MFB. *Science* **186**, 833–835.

Gebber, G. L., Taylor, D. G., and Weaver, L. C. (1973). Electrophysiological studies on organization of central vasopressor pathways. *Am. J. Physiol.* **224**, 470–481.

Geis, G. S., and Wurster, R. D. (1978). Localization of cardiac vagal preganglionic soma. *Soc. Neurosci. Abstr.* **4**, 20.

Gilbert, P. F. C., and Thach, W. T. (1977). Purkinje cell activity during motor learning. *Brain Res.* **128**, 309–328.

Gildenberg, P. L. (1969). Localization of a site of angiotensin vasopressor activity in the brain. *Physiologist* **12**, 235.

Gillis, R. A., and Williford, D. J. (1979). Evidence for involvement of a CNS GABAergic mechanism in reflex-induced vagal bradycardia in the cat. *Soc. Neurosci. Abstr.* **5**, 42.

Grant, G. (1962). Spinal course and somatotopically localized termination of the spinocerebellar tracts: An experimental study in cat. *Acta Physiol. Scand. Suppl.* **193**, 5–42.

Guertzenstein, P. G. (1973). Blood pressure effects obtained by drugs applied to the ventral surface of the brain stem. *J. Physiol.* **229**, 395–408.

Haas, H. L., Anderson, E. G., and Hösli, L. (1973). Histamine and metabolites: their effects and interactions with convulsants on brain stem neurons. *Brain Res.* **51**, 269–278.

Hellner, K., and von Baumgarten, R. (1961). Über ein Endigungsgebiet afferenter, kardiovasculärer Fasern des Nervus vagus im Rautenhirn der Katze. *Pfluegers Arch. Gesamte Physiol. Menschen Tiere* **273**, 223–224.

Hennemann, H. E., and Rubia, F. J. (1978). Vagal representation in the cerebellum of the cat. *Pfluegers Arch.* **375**, 119–123.

Henry, J. L., and Calaresu, F. R. (1972). Distribution of cardioacceleratory sites in intermediolateral nucleus of the cat. *Am. J. Physiol.* **222**, 700–704.

Henry, J. L., and Calaresu, F. R. (1974). Excitatory in inhibitory inputs from medullary nuclei projecting to spinal cardio-acceleratory neurons in the cat. *Exp. Brain Res.* **20**, 485–504.

Hilton, S. M., and Spyer, K. M. (1971). Participation of the anterior hypothalamus in the baroreceptor reflex. *J. Physiol. (London)* **218**, 271–293.

Hockman, C. H., Livingston, K. E. and Talesnik, J. (1970). Cerebellar modulation of reflex vagal bradycardia. *Brain Res.* **23**, 101–104.

Hoffer, B. J. (1965). The effects of stimulation of the cerebellum on the circulatory system. Ph.D. Thesis. Univ. of Rochester, Rochester, New York.

Hökfelt, T., Fuxe, K., Johansson, O., and Ljungdahl, Å. (1974). Pharmacohistochemical evidence of the existence of dopamine nerve terminals in the limbic cortex. *Eur. J. Pharmacol.* **25,** 108–112.

Humphrey, D. R. (1967). Neuronal activity in the medulla oblongata of cat evoked by stimulation of the carotid sinus nerve. *In* "Baroreceptors and Hypertension" (P. Kedzi, ed.), pp. 131–168. Pergamon, Oxford.

Johansson, O., Hökfelt, T., Elde, R. P., Schultzberg, M., and Terenius, L. (1978). Immunohistochemical distribution of enkephalin neurons. *In* "Advances in Biochemical Psychopharmacology, Vol. 18" (E. Costa and M. Trabucchi, eds.), pp. 51–70. Raven Press, New York.

Julius, S. (1976). Introduction. *In* "The Nervous System in Arterial Hypertension" (S. Julius and M. D. Esler, eds.), pp. xii–xvi. Thomas, Springfield, Illinois.

Katz, D. M., and Karten, H. J. (1979). The discrete anatomical localization of vagal aortic afferents within a catecholamine containing cell groups in the nucleus solitarius. *Brain Res.* **171,** 187–195.

Kawamura, H., Gunn, C. G., and Frohlich, E. D. (1978). Cardiovascular alteration by nucleus locus coeruleus in spontaneously hypertensive rats. *Brain Res.* **140,** 137–147.

Kennedy, P. R. (1978). The olive and central control of blood pressure. *Med. Hypotheses* **4,** 593–595.

Kerr, F. W. L. (1969). Preserved vagal visceromotor function following destruction of the dorsal motor nucleus. *J. Physiol. (London)* **202,** 755–769.

Korner, P. I. (1971). Integrative neural cardiovascular control. *Physiol. Rev.* **51,** 312–367.

Kumada, M., Dampney, R. A. L., and Reis, D. J. (1979). Profound hypotension and abolition of the vasomotor component of the cerebral ischemic response produced by restricted lesions of medulla oblongata in rabbit. *Circ. Res.* **45,** 63–70.

Kumada, M., and Nakajima, H. (1972). Field potentials evoked in rabbit brainstem by stimulation of the aortic nerve. *Am. J. Physiol.* **223,** 575–582.

Kuru, M., Koyama, Y., and Kurati, T. (1960). The bulbar vesico-relaxer center and the bulbosacral connections arising from it. *J. Comp. Neurol.* **113,** 365–388.

Laborde, J. V. (1888). Du noyau d'origine, dans le bulbe rachidien des fibres motorices ou cardiaques du nerf pneumogastrique, ou noyau cardiaque. *Arch. Physiol. Norm. Pathol.* **4,** 397–417.

Larson, B., Miller, S., and Oscarsson, O. (1969). A spinocerebellar climbing fibre path activated by the flexor reflex afferents from all four limbs. *J. Physiol. (London)* **203,** 641–649.

Laubie, M., Schmitt, H., and Drouillat, M. (1977). Central sites and mechanisms of the hypotensive and bradycardic effects of the narcotic analgesic agent fentanyl. *Naunyn-Schmiedebergs Arch. Exp. Pathol. Pharmakol.* **296,** 255–261.

Lipinski, J. F., Schaumburg, H. H., and Baldessarini, R. J. (1973). Regional distribution of histamine in the human brain. *Brain Res.* **52,** 403–408.

Lisander, B., and Martner, J. (1971). Interaction between the fastigial pressor response and the baroreceptor reflex. *Acta Physiol. Scand.* **83,** 505–514.

Löfving, B. (1961). Cardiovascular adjustments induced from the rostral cingulate gyrus. *Acta Physiol. Scand. Suppl.* **184,** 1–82.

Martner, J. (1975). Cerebellar influences on autonomic mechanisms: An experimental study in the cat with special reference to the fastigial nucleus. *Acta Physiol. Scand. Suppl.* **425,** 5–42.

McGeer, P. L., Eccles, J. C., and McGeer, E. G. (1978). Cholinergic neurons. *In* "Molecular Neurobiology of the Mammalian Brain," p. 160. Plenum, New York.

Middleton, S., Woolsey, C. N., and Rose, J. E. (1965). Electrocardiogram-related neural activity in medulla of cat. *Physiologist* **8,** 235.

Miskolczy, D. (1931). Über die endigungsweise der spino-cerebellaren bahnen. *Z. Anat. Entwicklungsgesch.* **96**, 537–542.

Miura, M., and Kitamura T. (1979). Postsynaptic potentials recorded from medullary neurones following stimulation of carotid sinus nerve. *Brain Res.* **162**, 261–272.

Miura, M., and Reis, D. J. (1969). Termination and secondary projections of carotid sinus nerve in the cat brain stem. *Am. J. Physiol.* **217**, 142–153.

Miura, M., and Reis, D. J. (1971). The paramedian reticular nucleus: a site of inhibitory interaction between projections from fastigial nucleus and carotid sinus nerve acting on blood pressure. *J. Physiol. (London)* **216**, 441–460.

Miura, M., and Reis, D. J. (1972). The role of the solitary and paramedian reticular nuclei in mediating cardiovascular reflex responses from carotid baro- and chemoreceptors. *J. Physiol. (London)* **223**, 525–548.

Mizuno, N., and Nakamura, Y. (1970). Direct hypothalamic projections to the locus coeruleus. *Brain Res.* **19**, 160–162.

Morest, D. K. (1967). Experimental study of the projections of the nucleus of the tractus solitarius and the area postrema in the cat. *J. Comp. Neurol.* **130**, 277–299.

Moruzzi, G. (1940). Paleocerebellar inhibition of vasomotor and respiratory carotid sinus reflexes. *J. Neurophysiol.* **3**, 20–32.

Moruzzi, G. (1950). "Problems in Cerebellar Physiology." Thomas, Springfield, Illinois.

Nakamura, S. (1975). Two types of inhibitory effects upon brain stem reticular neurons by low frequency stimulation of raphé nucleus in the rat. *Brain Res.* **93**, 140–144.

Nara, Y., Yamori, Y., and Lovenberg, W. (1978). Effect of dietary taurine on blood pressure in spontaneously hypertensive rats. *Biochem. Pharmacol.* **27**, 2689–2692.

Neumayr, R. J., Hare, B. D., and Franz, D. N. (1974). Evidence for bulbospinal control of sympathetic preganglionic neurons by monoaminergic pathways. *Life Sci.* **14**, 793–806.

Nosaka, S., Yamamoto, T., and Yasunaga, K. (1979). Localization of vagal cardioinhibitory preganglionic neurons within rat brain stem. *J. Comp. Neurol.* **186**, 79–92.

Norris, R. D., Foreman, R. D., and Wurster, R. D. (1974). Responses of the canine heart to stimulation of the first five ventral thoracic roots. *Am. J. Physiol.* **227**, 9–12.

Ogawa, M. (1978). Interaction between noradrenergic and serotonergic mechanisms on the central regulation of blood pressure in the rat: a study using experimental central hypertension produced by chemical lesions of the locus coeruleus. *Jpn. Circ. J.* **42**, 581–597.

Ogawa, M., Fujita, Y., Niwa, M., Takami, N., and Ozaki, M. (1977). An experimental central noradrenergic hypertension. *Jpn. Circ. J.* **41**, 883–885.

Owsjannikow, P. (1871). Die tonischen und reflectorischen centren der gefassnerven. *Ber. Verh. Sächs Akad. Wiss., Leipzig Math.–Phys. Kl.* **23**, 135–147.

Pagani, M., Schwartz, P. J., Banks, R., Lombardi, F., and Malliani, A. (1974). Reflex responses of sympathetic preganglionic neurones initiated by different cardiovascular receptors in spinal animals. *Brain Res.* **68**, 215–226.

Palkovits, M., and L. Záborsky (1977). Neuroanatomy of central cardiovascular control. Nucleus tractus solitarii: Afferent and efferent neuronal connections in relation to the baroreceptor reflex arc. *In* "Progress Brain Research, Vol. 47, Hypertension and Brain Mechanisms" (W. De Jong and A. P. Shapiro, eds.), pp. 9–34. Elsevier, Amsterdam.

Precht, W., Schwindt, P. C., and Baker, R. (1973). Removal of vestibular commissural inhibition by antagonists of GABA and glycine. *Brain Res.* **62**, 222–226.

Ranson, S. W., and Billingsley, P. R. (1916). Afferent spinal paths and the vasomotor reflexes. Studies in vasomotor reflex arcs VI. *Am. J. Physiol.* **42,** 16–35.

Reis, D. J. (1972). Central neural mechanisms governing the circulation with particular reference to the lower brain stem and cerebellum. *In* "Neural and Psychological Mechanisms in Cardiovascular Disease" (A. Zanchetti, ed.), pp. 255–280. Casa Editrice, Milan.

Reis, D. J., and Cuénod, M. (1965). Central neural regulation of carotid barocepter reflexes in the cat. *Am. J. Physiol.* **209,** 1267–1277.

Saavedra, J. M., Palkovits, M., Brownstein, M. J., and Axelrod, J. (1974). Serontonin distribution in the nuclei of the rat hypothalamus and preoptic region. *Brain Res.* **77,** 157–165.

Sato, A. (1975). Central organization of the autonomic nervous system. *Brain Res.* **87,** 137–448.

Satoh, M., Akaike, A., and Takagi, H. (1979). Excitation by morphine and enkephalin of single neurons of nucleus reticularis paragigantocellularis in the rat: a probable mechanism of analgesic action of opioids. *Brain Res.* **169,** 406–410.

Schramm, L. P., Howland, E. W., McKenna, K. E., and Barton, G. N. (1978). Splanchnic evoked responses and silent periods elicited from spinal cord of rat. *Fed. Proc. Fed. Am. Soc. Exp. Biol.* **37,** 744.

Schramm, L. P., Gunther, H. J., McKenna, K. E., and Barton, G. N. (1979a). Sympathetic hyperactivity and hypertension in adult spontaneously hypertensive rats despite early dorsolateral funicular lesions. *Brain Res.* **167,** 402–407.

Schramm, L. P., Howland, E. W., McKenna, K. E., and Barton, G. N. (1979b). Spinal pathways mediating splanchnic sympathetic excitation and sympathetic silent periods in the rat. *Brain Res.* **167,** 396–401.

Schwartz, J.-C. (1975). Minireview: Histamine as a transmitter in brain. *Life Sci.* **17,** 503–518.

Schwartz, J.-C. (1977). Histaminergic mechanisms in brain. *Annu. Rev. Pharmacol. Toxicol.* **17,** 325–339.

Sheridan, G., and Reis, D. J. (1972). Effects of cerebellar ablation on regional distribution of cardiac output in cat. *Brain Res.* **45,** 260–265.

Sjoerdsma, A. (1977). Central action as a key to past and future therapy of hypertension. *In* "Progress in Brain Research, Vol. 47, Hypertension and Brain Mechanisms" (W. De Jong, A. P. Provoost and A. P. Shapiro, eds.), pp. 1–5. Elsevier, Amsterdam.

Smirnov, K. A., and Potekhina, T. L. (1974). Localization and properties of reticulospinal neurons with axons descending in the dorsolateral parts of the spinal cord lateral funiculi. *Neurophysiology (Engl. Transl.)* **6,** 266–272.

Smith, O. A. (1974). Reflex and central mechanisms involved in the control of the heart and circulation. *Annu. Rev. Physiol.* **36,** 93–124.

Smith, O. A., and Clarke, N. P. (1964). Central autonomic pathways. A study in functional neuroanatomy. *J. Comp. Neurol.* **122,** 399–406.

Smith, O. A., Jr., and Nathan, M. A. (1966). Inhibition of the carotid sinus reflex by stimulation of the inferior olive. *Science* **154,** 674–675.

Smits, J. F. M., Van Essen, H., and Struyker-Boudier, A. J. (1978). Serotonin-mediated cardiovascular responses to electrical stimulation of the raphe nuclei in the rat. *Life Sci.* **23,** 173–178.

Snider, R. S. (1936). Alterations which occur in mossy terminals of the cerebellum following transection of brachium pontis. *J. Comp. Neurol.* **64,** 417–435.

Snyder, D. W., Boccagno, J. A., and Antonaccio, M. J. (1979). Brainstem areas mediating the hypotensive effects of muscimol. *Soc. Neurosci. Abstr.* **5,** 51.

Sobusiak, T., Zinny, R., and Zabel, J. (1972). Comparative pattern of the primary afferent projection from the VIIIth, IXth, and Xth cranial nerves to the accessory cuneate nucleus. *Anat. Anz.* **131,** 248–258.

Spring, D. D., and Haigler, H. J. (1979). Effects of morphine (MS), methionine-enkephalin (ME), and substance P (SP) on neuronal firing in the nucleus reticularis gigantocellularis (NRGc) of the rat. *Soc. Neurosci. Abstr.* **5,** 572.

Starke, K., Endo, T., and Taube, H. D. (1976). Central noradrenergic mechanisms of neurotransmission. *In* "Regulation of Blood Pressure by the Central Nervous System" (G. Onesti, M. Fernandes, and K. E. Kim, eds.), pp. 21–34. Grune and Stratton, New York.

Strahlendorf, H. K., Strahlendorf, J. C., and Barnes, C. D. (1980). Endorphin mediated inhibition of locus coeruleus neurons. *Brain Res.* (in press).

Strahlendorf, J. C., Strahlendorf, H. K., and Barnes, C. D. (1979). Modulation of cerebellar neuronal activity by raphe stimulation. *Brain Res.* **169,** 565–569.

Sugimoto, T., Itoh, K., Mizuno, N., Nomura, S., and Konishi, A. (1979). The site of origin of cardiac preganglionic fibers of the vagus nerve: An HRP study in cat. *Neurosci. Lett.* (in press).

Szentagothai, J., and Rajkovits, K. (1959). Über den ursprung der kletterfasern des kleinhirns. *Z. Anat. Entwicklungsgesch* **121,** 130–141.

Takeuchi, T., and Manning, J. W. (1973). Hypothalamic mediation of sinus baroreceptor-evoked muscle cholinergic dilator response. *Am. J. Physiol.* **224,** 1280–1287.

Tangri, K. K., Jain, I. P., and Bhargava, K. P. (1977). Role of central cholinoceptors in cardiovascular regulation. *In* "Progress Brain Research, Vol. 47, Hypertension and Brain Mechanisms" (W. De Jong, A. P. Provoost and A. P. Shapiro, eds.), pp. 123–135. Elsevier, Amsterdam.

Taylor, K. M., Geller, E., and Snyder, S. H. (1972). Regional localization of histamine and histidine in the brain of the Rhesus monkey. *Brain Res.* **41,** 171–179.

Taylor, K. M., and Snyder, S. H. (1971). Histamine in the rat brain: sensitive assay of endogenous levels, formation *in vivo* and lowering by inhibitors of histidine decarboxylase. *J. Pharmacol. Exp. Ther.* **179,** 619–633.

Thomas, M. R., and Calaresu, F. R. (1974). Localization and function of medullary sites mediating vagal bradycardia in the cat. *Am. J. Physiol.* **226,** 1344–1349.

Ward, D. G., and Gunn, C. G. (1976). Locus coeruleus complex: elicitation of a pressor response and a brain stem region necessary for its occurrence. *Brain Res.* **107,** 401–406.

Wijnen, H. J. L. M., DeKloet, E. R., and Versteeg, D. H. G. (1978). Differences in regional brain catecholamine metabolism after a decrease in blood pressure. *Life Sci.* **23,** 2587–2592.

Wurster, R. D. (1977). Spinal sympathetic control of the heart. *In* "Neural Regulation of the Heart" (Walter C. Randall, ed.), pp. 213–246. Oxford Univ. Press, London and New York.

Zandberg, P., and De Jong, W. (1977). Localization of catecholaminergic receptor sites in the nucleus tractus solitarii involved in the regulation of arterial blood pressure. *In* "Progress in Brain Research, Vol. 47, Hypertension and Brain Mechanisms" (W. De Jong, A. P. Provoost, and A. P. Shapiro, eds.), pp. 117–122. Elsevier, Amsterdam.

3

Bulbospinal Control of Sympathetic Nerve Discharge

Gerard L. Gebber

I. INTRODUCTION

The purpose of this chapter is to expose the reader to the most basic problems relating to brain stem and spinal control of the discharges of preganglionic sympathetic neurons. An exhaustive review of the literature is not provided; rather, the chapter is based primarily on electrophysiological data collected in my laboratory since 1972. Many of the experiments have been performed on sympathetic nerves which are contained in cardiovascular pathways. Consequently, it is probable that at

NEURAL CONTROL OF CIRCULATION

least some of the conclusions can be related to central sympathetic networks which govern the vasculature and heart. After a brief historical review, several questions are considered. First, how are the background discharges in sympathetic nerves generated? Second, how is activity in brain stem circuits transmitted to the preganglionic sympathetic neurons of the spinal cord? Third, what are the sites of baroreceptor-induced sympathoinhibition? Fourth, what are the characteristics of the final common pathway, i.e., the preganglionic sympathetic neuron? Fifth, do spinal sympathetic networks act primarily as relay stations or as integrating circuits? Finally, problems related to the identification of the individual components of brain stem and spinal circuits responsible for the background discharges of preganglionic sympathetic neurons are discussed.

II. HISTORICAL OVERVIEW

Over 100 years ago, Bernard (1863) demonstrated that transection of the cervical spinal cord led to a pronounced fall in blood pressure. The implications of this experiment are clear: there is a neurogenic component for the support of resting blood pressure. This support, of course, arises from the background discharges in preganglionic sympathetic neurons. Moreover, the experiments of Bernard indicate that the background discharges in sympathetic nerves arise, for the most part, as the consequence of activity generated in neural networks located above the level of spinal transection, i.e., the brain.

In the early 1870s, Dittmar (1873) and Owsjannikow (1871) defined those regions of the brain responsible for generating the background discharges in sympathetic nerves. Their approach was to study the effects on blood pressure produced by serial transections of the brain stem in the rabbit. Transection of the neuraxis above the caudal one-third of the pons produced very little change in blood pressure. Thus, it was assumed that the forebrain was not important in maintaining blood pressure, at least in the anesthetized animal. Transections made more caudally revealed that the basal discharges of sympathetic nerves arose from networks located in the caudal one-third of the pons and the rostral two-thirds of the medulla (i.e., between sections A and C in Fig. 1). This point was demonstrated directly with recordings made from the cervical and inferior cardiac sympathetic nerves in a later study by Alexander (1946).

Almost 50 years elapsed before Ranson and Billingsley (1916) began their studies on the location of cardiovascular reactive sites in the brain

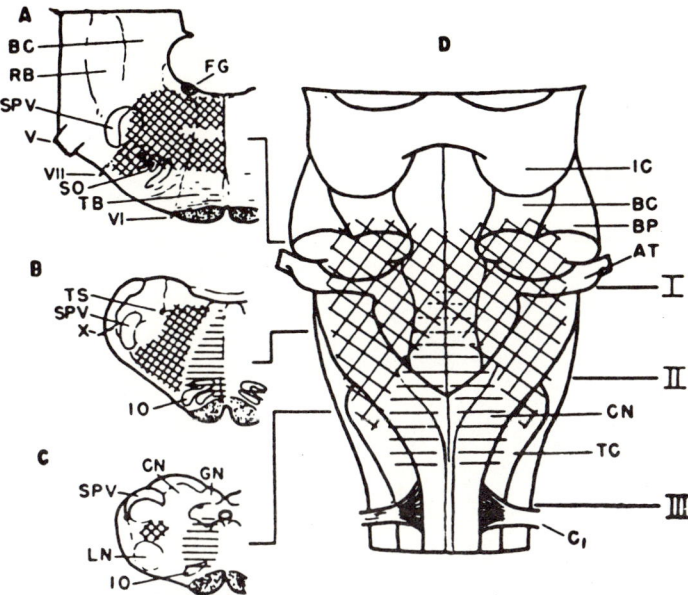

Fig. 1. Pressor and depressor regions of brain stem in the cat. Pressor region indicated by cross-hatching, depressor region by horizontal ruling. (A)–(C) Frontal sections through medulla at levels indicated by guide lines to D. (D) Pressor and depressor regions projected onto dorsal surface of brain stem. I, II, III in D are levels of transection discussed by Alexander (1946). AT, auditory tubercle; BC, brachium conjunctiva; BP, brachium pontis; C_1, first cervical nerve; CN, cuneate nucleus; FG, facial genu; GN, gracile nucleus; IC, inferior colliculus; IO, inferior olivary nucleus; LN, lateral reticular nucleus; RB, restiform body; SO, superior olivary nucleus; SPV, spinal trigeminal tract; TB, trapezoid body; TC, tuberculum cinereum; TS, tractus solitarius; V, VI, VII, corresponding cranial nerves. (From Alexander, 1946, with permission of *J. Neurophysiology*.)

stem. They found two discrete areas on the dorsal surface of the medulla (i.e., the floor of the fourth ventricle) from which blood pressure could be changed with electrical stimulation. A decrease in blood pressure (later shown to be due primarily to inhibition of sympathetic nerve traffic) could be elicited from a medial medullary point near the obex. An increase in blood pressure was produced by stimulation of an area somewhat lateral and rostral to the depressor site. Although Ranson and Billingsley were careful not to attribute their results to the activation of functionally discrete and anatomically circumscribed "centers"; others were not so cautious in their interpretation; therefore, the misconception of discrete cardiovascular "centers" arose.

The pendulum swung to the other extreme in 1939. Using the Horsley–Clarke stereotaxic technique, Wang and Ranson (1939a) reexplored the brain stem for cardiovascular reactive sites. It is important to note that the depths of the brain stem, as well as the dorsal surface, were electrically stimulated in this study. As shown in Fig. 1B, the pressor and depressor points found earlier on the dorsal surface of the medulla by Ranson and Billingsley (1916) were not discrete "centers" but rather, the apexes of two triangles, which extended almost to the ventral surface of the brain stem through the reticular formation. Decreases in blood pressure were most often produced by stimulation of the medial reticular formation. Increases in blood pressure were usually elicited by stimulation of the periventricular gray and lateral reticular formation. Anatomists and physiologists took a dim view of the reticular formation in the 1930s; it was considered haphazardly organized. Primarily on the basis of this erroneous assumption (see reviews in Brodal, 1957; Scheibel and Scheibel, 1958), the results of Wang and Ranson were interpreted as indicating that brain stem cardiovascular networks were diffuse in their organization. This concept, which still appears in many textbooks, will be challenged in this chapter.

The studies discussed thus far were unquestionably important in defining the general region of the brain stem responsible for the background discharges in sympathetic nerves and the location of central cardiovascular reactive sites. Our knowledge of the central control of sympathetic nerve discharge, however, remained largely incomplete. For instance, the transection experiments did not provide information on the intrinsic organization of those brain-stem circuits responsible for generating the background discharges of preganglionic sympathetic neurons. Furthermore, the stimulation experiments failed to reveal which element (afferent, internuncial, or bulbospinal) of a pathway was activated in any given instance. These experiments also did not deal with the question of how many different sympathoexcitatory and sympathoinhibitory pathways exist. These problems, among others, are discussed in the following sections.

III. CURRENT RESEARCH TOPICS

A. The Generating System Responsible for Basal Sympathetic Nerve Discharge

Adrian *et al.* (1932) were first to record and characterize the background discharges in sympathetic nerve bundles. These discharges exhibit one or a combination of three different rhythmic (i.e., periodic) components. Sympathetic nerve discharge is usually synchronized into bursts which are locked in a 1:1 relation to the cardiac cycle. As shown in Fig. 2, the amplitude of the cardiac-related bursts of sympathetic nerve

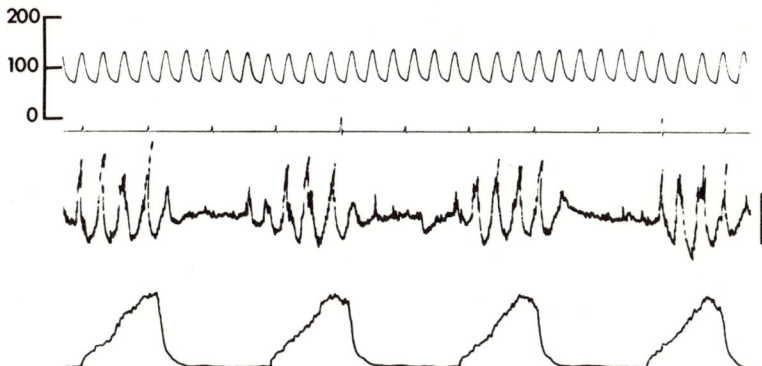

Fig. 2. Rhythmic components in sympathetic nerve discharge of a vagotomized cat. Top trace shows blood pressure (mmHg). Middle trace shows background discharges of external carotid, postganglionic sympathetic nerve (negativity recorded as an upward deflection in this and in subsequent figures; preamplifier bandpass was 1–1000 Hz). Bottom trace shows RC integrated (time constant 0.05 sec), phrenic nerve discharge (inspiration recorded as an upward deflection). Time base (below blood pressure) is 1 sec per division. Vertical calibration is 40 μv and applies to sympathetic nerve discharge. (From Barman and Gebber, 1976, with permission of *Am. J. Physiology*.)

activity often waxes and wanes with the period of the respiratory cycle (as monitored from phrenic nerve discharge). Thus, sympathetic nerve discharge contains a respiratory-related periodicity. The discharges of sympathetic nerve bundles are almost always greatest in amplitude during the inspiratory phase of the respiratory cycle in vagotomized cats. As will be discussed in detail subsequently, a more rapid periodicity (8–12 cps) sometimes is observed in place of, or in combination with, the cardiac-related rhythm.

Perhaps the most basic problem to be discussed concerns the origin of the background discharges in sympathetic nerves. One of the keys to this problem is understanding how the discharges of numerous preganglionic sympathetic neurons are synchronized into cardiac-related, respiratory-related and 8–12 cps bursts. The traditional view assumes that the basal discharges of brain-stem neurons, which provide driving inputs to preganglionic sympathetic neurons, are generated randomly (i.e., the random generation theory). This theory implies that central sympathetic networks, responsible for the background discharges in preganglionic sympathetic neurons, are diffusely organized in that they lack internal oscillating circuits. The basics of the random generation theory follow. First, factors such as the local chemical environment (pH, P_{CO_2}, P_{O_2}) and converging asynchronous inputs from sensory pathways are believed to generate random discharges in brain-stem reticular neurons in sympatho-excitatory networks. Second, the randomly generated discharges of numerous brain stem reticular neurons are believed to be synchronized by specialized inputs to produce the cardiac- and respiratory-related rhythms. The cardiac-related rhythm in sympathetic nerve discharge is believed to result as the simple consequence of the baroreceptor reflexes (Adrian et al., 1932; Cohen and Gootman, 1970; Heymans and Neil, 1958). That is, increased baroreceptor nerve discharge during systole supposedly causes a delayed inhibition of sympathetic nerve activity, while the removal of inhibition during diastole leads to an increase in sympathetic nerve discharge. It is also assumed that the brain-stem respiratory oscillator imposes its rhythm on the diffusely organized central sympathetic network (Cohen and Gootman, 1970; Koizumi et al., 1971). Thus, the random generation theory attributes the rhythms in sympathetic nerve discharge to sources extrinsic to the brain-stem generating system.

The first crack in the random generation theory occurred with the experiments of Cohen and Gootman (1970) and Green and Heffron (1967). These investigators observed an 8–12 cps periodicity in the discharges of preganglionic and postganglionic sympathetic nerve bundles, which usually was not locked to the phases of the cardiac cycle. Thus, it became apparent that central sympathetic networks were inherently capable of synchronizing the discharges of populations of preganglionic sympathetic neurons. This realization constitutes a marked departure from the random generation theory. Sympathetic nerve rhythms intrinsic to the brain stem and/or spinal cord imply the existence of well-organized central networks containing either pacemaker neurons or oscillating circuits (most likely the latter, in my opinion). In this case, rhythms in sympathetic nerve discharge would be representative of the fundamental organization of those central circuits that generate the background activity of the system (i.e., the intrinsic oscillator theory).

Experiments performed on cats in our laboratory have extended the intrinsic oscillator theory to the cardiac- and respiratory-related periodicities. We believe that both rhythms are generated intrinsically in brain-stem networks rather than by periodically occurring extrinsic inputs from the baroreceptor nerves and the respiratory oscillator. Considering the cardiac-related rhythm (3–5 cps periodicity) in sympathetic nerve discharge, we have found that:

(1) Bilateral section of the carotid sinus, aortic depressor, and vagus nerves did not eliminate the 3–5 cps periodicity (Taylor and Gebber, 1975). Rather, baroreceptor denervation simply unlocked the 1:1 relation between the 3–5 cps bursts in sympathetic nerve discharge and the cardiac cycle. The ratio of sympathetic nerve bursts per cardiac cycle was greater than 1, following baroreceptor denervation.

(2) It was possible to produce dramatic shifts in the phase relations between baroreceptor nerve activity and sympathetic nerve discharge by slowing the heart rate (Gebber, 1976). This observation also failed to support the notion that the cardiac-related periodicity was the simple consequence of the waxing and waning of baroreceptor nerve discharge. If this were the case, then the phase relations between sympathetic and baroreceptor nerve discharges should have been independent of the heart rate.

(3) Single shocks applied to the baroreceptor nerves early in the cardiac cycle aborted one complete cycle of sympathetic nerve discharge (Taylor and Gebber, 1975).

These results led us to conclude that the cardiac-related periodicity in sympathetic nerve discharge is representative of a rhythm of central origin. The rhythm is generated in the brain stem, since it could not be demonstrated in residual sympathetic nerve discharge after transection of the high cervical spinal cord (McCall and Gebber, 1975), and because it persisted after midcollicular decerebration (S. M. Barman and G. L. Gebber, unpublished observations). Furthermore, we concluded that, rather than creating the rhythm, the function of the baroreceptor reflexes was to entrain the centrally generated rhythm in a 1:1 relation to the cardiac cycle for the purpose of limiting the frequency of the brain-stem oscillating circuit.

Our experiments also revealed that the slow rhythm in sympathetic nerve discharge of the vagotomized cat is generated by a brain-stem oscillator distinct from that responsible for the rhythmic discharges of respiratory neurons. The slow sympathetic and respiratory oscillators, however, are normally entrained to each other in some as-yet undefined way. The independent oscillator hypothesis for the slow sympathetic rhythm is based on the following observations, which can be found in two of our recent publications (Barman and Gebber, 1976; Gebber and Barman, 1977). First, changes in respiratory rate (as monitored from the phrenic nerve in paralyzed, vagotomized, and artificially ventilated cats) were accompanied by dramatic shifts in the phase relations between phrenic and sympathetic nerve activity. This observation makes it difficult to accept the view that the slow periodicity in sympathetic nerve discharge results from direct coupling between one of the components of the brain-stem respiratory oscillator and a diffusely organized central sympathetic network (i.e., extrinsic imposition of the rhythm). If such was the case, then the phase relations between the discharges of the sympathetic nerves and the phrenic nerve should have been independent of the respiratory rate. Second, we found that slow oscillations in sympathetic and phrenic nerve discharges were not always locked in a 1:1 relation. Instances of

3:2 and 1:2 locking of sympathetic and phrenic nerve discharges were observed. Finally, we demonstrated that the slow periodic component in sympathetic nerve discharge often persisted when the rhythmic discharges of the phrenic nerve disappeared during hypocapnia, a condition produced by increasing the rate of artificial ventilation. It would be impossible to attribute the genesis of the slow sympathetic rhythm directly to periodic input from the brain-stem respiratory oscillator, under these conditions. Thus, we postulated the existence of a slow sympathetic oscillator located in the brain stem, whose elements are less apt to lose their rhythmic discharge pattern during hypocapnia than are those components of the respiratory oscillator.

As already mentioned, Cohen and Gootman (1970) and Green and Heffron (1967) observed an 8–12 cps periodicity in the discharges of whole sympathetic nerves in cats and dogs with intact neuraxes. More recent experiments performed in our laboratory (McCall and Gebber, 1975) demonstrated that this rhythm exists in sympathetic nerve discharge in the high spinal cat under hypercapnic conditions (see Panel D in Fig. 3). Thus, it is apparent that spinal, as well as brain-stem networks, are inherently capable of synchronizing the discharges of populations of preganglionic sympathetic neurons.

In summary, the background discharges of preganglionic sympathetic neurons are generated in at least three distinct oscillating circuits located in the brain stem and spinal cord. Elucidation of the intrinsic organization of each circuit and the interactions between circuits awaits recording experiments at the level of the single cell. Nevertheless, it is apparent that the classic concept of a diffusely and primitively organized, central sympathetic network has not passed the test of time.

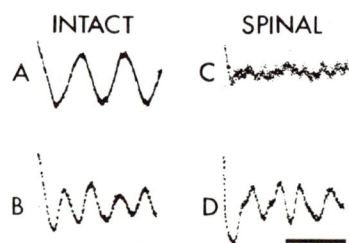

Fig. 3. Autocorrelograms of renal sympathetic nerve discharge in cats with intact neuraxes or with high spinal transection. Autocorrelograms from two intact cats show ≅3 cps (A), and ≅10 cps (B) periodic components. Autocorrelograms from a high spinal cat under resting conditions (C), and during hypercapnia (D). Address bin was 2 msec in A–D. Sample run was 4 min in A–C and 3 min in D. Autocorrelogram D was constructed from data obtained during six, 30-sec periods of asphyxia. Horizontal calibration is 500 msec for A, and 250 msec for B–D. (From McCall and Gebber, 1975, with permission of *Brain Research*.)

B. Parallel Arrangement of Bulbospinal
Sympathoexcitatory Pathways

Once impulses are generated within brain stem oscillating circuits, they must be successfully transmitted to preganglionic sympathetic neurons in the intermediolateral nucleus of the thoraco-lumbar spinal cord. A major question concerning this process is whether driving inputs from the brain to a given preganglionic sympathetic neuron are mediated over more than one pathway. As discussed by Peiss (1965), a parallel arrangement of pathways would allow for independent control of the preganglionic sympathetic neuron by different brain regions. This possibility was first postulated for the medulla and hypothalamus by Wang and Ranson (1939b). Electrophysiological experiments performed in our laboratory in 1973 (Gebber *et al.,* 1973; Snyder and Gebber, 1973) demonstrated that preganglionic sympathetic neurons receive parallel driving inputs from the brain and that transmission in each of two distinct sympathoexcitatory pathways is differentially controlled by the baroreceptor reflexes.

Two response types were elicited in the external carotid, postganglionic sympathetic nerve of the cat when single shocks or short trains of pulses were applied to pressor sites in the lateral hypothalamus, medulla, or dorsolateral funiculus of the cervical spinal cord. Examples of each response type elicited by medullary stimulation are shown in Fig. 4. One response type had long onset latencies (>50 msec), low following frequencies, and was inhibited by baroreceptor reflex activation. This response type was termed the baroreceptor-sensitive response (traces A1, A2, B1, and B2 in Fig. 4). The second response type (traces A4 and B3 in Fig. 4) had shorter onset latencies, followed higher frequencies of stimulation, and could not be inhibited (even when elicited by hypothalamic stimulation) by baroreceptor reflex activation. Postganglionic nerve discharges with these characteristics were termed baroreceptor-insensitive responses. Although both response types were observed on stimulation of some medullary pressor sites (trace A3 in Fig. 4), the baroreceptor-insensitive response was elicited primarily from nucleus reticularis ventralis, while the baroreceptor-sensitive postganglionic discharge was evoked from a much wider area of the medulla; including the periventricular gray, nucleus reticularis parvocellularis, and nucleus reticularis ventralis (Fig. 4). In a subsequent study (Taylor and Gebber, 1973), we demonstrated that the pathways responsible for the baroreceptor-sensitive and -insensitive discharges of the external carotid postganglionic nerve converged onto the same preganglionic neurons. This observation reinforced our view that both the short-latency and long-latency pathways subserved the same function (presumably vasopressor).

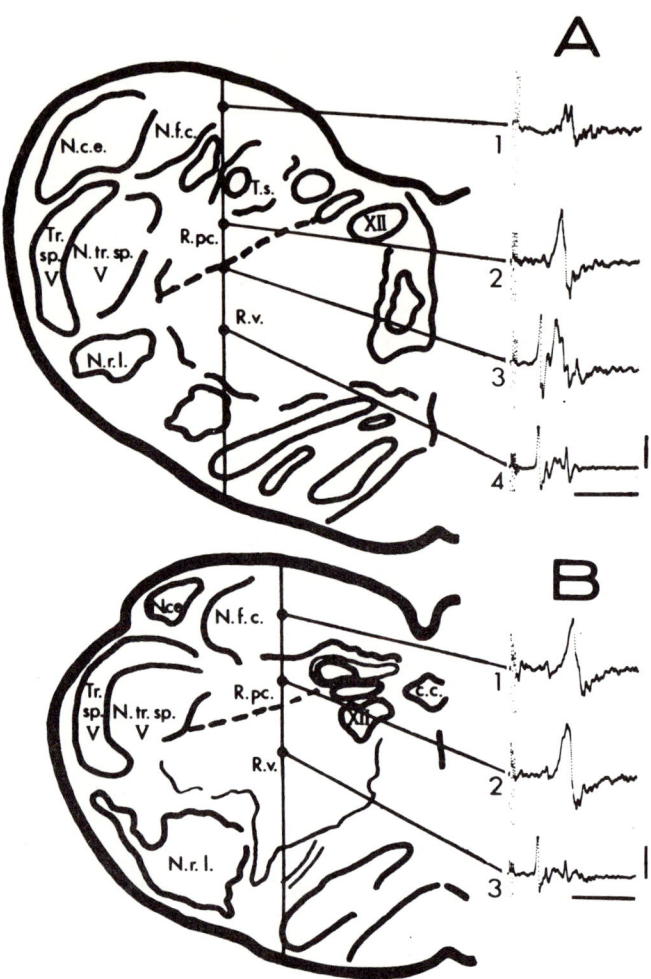

Fig. 4. Representative responses evoked in external carotid, postganglionic sympathetic nerve by stimulation of ipsilateral medulla of a decerebrate, unanesthetized cat. Ten millisecond trains of three pulses (10 V; 0.5 msec; 300 Hz) were applied to medullary pressor sites, once every sec. Each potential is a sum of 64 trials. (A) a frontal section about 2 mm rostral to obex. (B) a section about 1 mm caudal to obex. Horizontal calibration is 100 msec. Vertical calibration is 532 μV. c.c., central canal; N.c.e., external cuneate nucleus; N.f.c., nucleus cuneatus; N.r.l., lateral reticular nucleus; N.tr.sp.V, spinal nucleus of trigeminal nerve; R.pc., nucleus reticularis parvocellularis; R.v., nucleus reticularis ventralis; Tr.sp.V, spinal tract of trigeminal nerve; T.s., tractus solitarius; XII, motor nucleus of hypoglossal nerve. (From Gebber *et al.*, 1973, with permission of *Am. J. Physiology.*)

The long-latency pathway probably is involved in mediating the background discharges in sympathetic nerves. In this regard, Snyder and Gebber (1973) demonstrated that basal activity and long-latency-evoked potentials in the external carotid postganglionic nerve were equally sensitive to inhibition by baroreceptor reflex activation. The short-latency pathway was not tonically active under the conditions of our experiments with anesthetized cats. This conclusion is based on the observations that (1) short-latency postganglionic responses, elicited by stimulation of pressor sites as far rostral as the hypothalamus, could not be blocked during baroreceptor reflex activation; and (2) basal discharges in sympathetic nerves can be completely inhibited upon baroreceptor reflex activation. Future investigations should deal with the possibility that the short-latency pressor pathway plays a role in mediating phasic cardiovascular changes, perhaps of the type seen during the defense reaction.

C. Sites of Sympathoinhibition of Baroreceptor Reflex Origin

The nucleus of the tractus solitarius in the medulla is the primary site of termination of baroreceptor afferents of the carotid sinus and aortic depressor nerves (Miura and Reis, 1969; Seller and Illert, 1969). Neurons within this nucleus, in turn, send their axons to various brain-stem, forebrain, and spinal regions (Loewy and Burton, 1977; Miura and Reis, 1969; Palkovits and Zaborszky, 1977; Ricardo and Koh, 1977). Until recently, it was casually assumed that sympathoinhibition of baroreceptor reflex origin took place in the medulla. However, it is now known that transmission in sympathoexcitatory pathways can be interrupted by baroreceptor reflex activation, both at spinal and brain-stem levels.

Using computer summation, Taylor and Gebber (1975) studied the temporal characteristics of sympathoinhibition produced by single shocks or 5-msec trains of three pulses applied to a baroreceptor nerve or to intramedullary components of the baroreceptor reflex arc in the cat. Inhibition of the background discharges of the preganglionic splanchnic and postganglionic renal sympathetic nerves was displayed as a positive potential by the computer. Positive potentials result from intervals of decreased sympathetic nerve discharge time-locked to the stimulus. As shown in Fig. 5, early and late positive potentials were observed with trains of stimuli, while only the late period of inhibition was evident following single-shock stimulation. The onset of the early positive potential on the splanchnic nerve was $\cong 30$ msec, while that of the late positive potential was $\cong 100$ msec. The early positive potential lasted

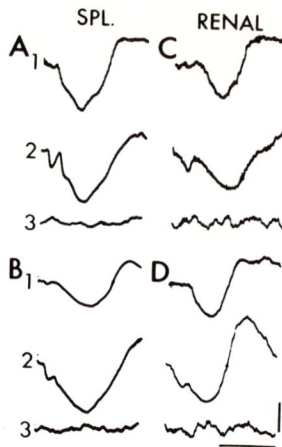

Fig. 5. Computer-summed traces (64 trials) of preganglionic splanchnic and post-ganglionic renal, sympathetic nerve positive potentials evoked by stimulation of paramedian reticular nucleus. A single shock or a 5 msec train of three pulses was applied once every 2 sec to the medullary site. A_1–D_1: positivity evoked by single shock stimulation. Each trace is from a different cat. A_2–D_2: positivity evoked in the same cats by trains of pulses. A_3–D_3: sum of 64 computer sweeps triggered in the same cats by dummy pulses. Horizontal calibration is 250 msec. Vertical calibration is 133 μV for A_1–A_3, 267 μV for B_1–B_3 and C_1–C_3, and 533 μV for D_1–D_3. (From Taylor and Gebber, 1975, with permission of *Am. J. Physiology*.)

$\cong$70 msec, while the late positive potential had a duration of $\cong$300 msec. Importantly, splanchnic nerve discharges, produced by stimuli applied to descending pressor tracts in the dorsolateral funiculus of the cervical spinal cord, were blocked during the time course of the early positive potential, but not during that of the late positive potential (Fig. 6). This observation led to the conclusion that the early period of inhibition of background sympathetic nerve discharge occurred in the spinal cord, while the late phase of inhibition occurred at a supraspinal level (i.e., at a site rostral to the point of activation of descending bulbospinal tracts in the cervical spinal cord). Both phases of inhibition were unaltered by midcollicular decerebration. Thus, forebrain loops in the baroreceptor reflex arc (Spyer, 1972; Thomas and Calaresu, 1972) are not critical for sympathoinhibition induced by an increase in baroreceptor afferent discharge. In summary, baroreceptor-induced sympathoinhibition is mediated both at spinal and at brain-stem levels. The organization of the bulbospinal inhibitory pathway is discussed in Section III,F.

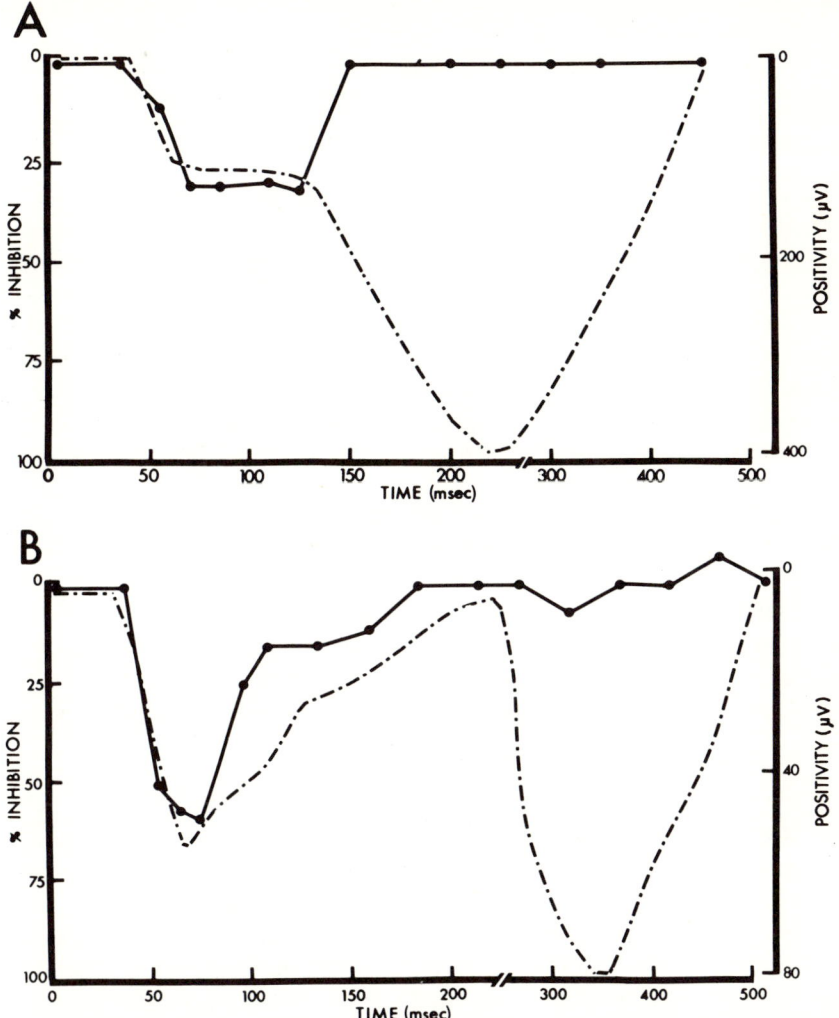

Fig. 6. Comparison of time course of computer-summed positivity, evoked by stimulation (5 msec trains of three pulses) of paramedian reticular nucleus in medulla, with that of inhibition of computer-summed splanchnic nerve response, elicited by a 10 msec train of three pulses applied to descending spinal pressor tracts in two cats (A and B). Dot-dash lines denote time course of positivity. Amplitude (μV) is plotted against time (msec) after stimuli were applied to depressor site in paramedian reticular nucleus. Solid lines denote time course of inhibition of splanchnic nerve discharge evoked by stimulation of descending spinal pressor site. Percent inhibition is plotted against the interval (msec) between paramedian stimulation and the onset of spinal → splanchnic nerve discharge. Curve was constructed by varying the interval between stimuli applied to the medulla and spinal cord. Percent inhibition was calculated on the basis of peak amplitude of control, spinal → splanchnic nerve discharge. (From Taylor and Gebber, 1975, with permisison of *Am. J. Physiology*.)

D. The Final Common Pathway

There is ample reason to believe that individual preganglionic sympathetic neurons in vasopressor pathways serve as the final common pathway for impulses arriving from all levels of the neuraxis and periphery. Taylor and Gebber (1973) demonstrated that individual preganglionic sympathetic neurons in the cat thoracic spinal cord could be activated by stimulation of widely separated medullary pressor sites, located in the reticular formation and periventricular gray. Moreover, the same preganglionic unit exhibited baroreceptor-sensitive and -insensitive discharges upon stimulation of the medullary pressor region. In addition, Seller (1973) noted that individual preganglionic sympathetic neurons receive converging excitatory inputs from the brain stem and somatic afferent nerves.

More recently, R. McCall and G. L. Gebber (unpublished observations) noted that individual preganglionic fibers, teased from the cervical sympathetic nerve in the cat, can exhibit all three of the periodicities commonly observed in the discharges of whole sympathetic nerve bundles. As shown in Fig. 7, the autocorrelograms of the discharges of unit A show a combination of a rapid rhythm with the period of the cardiac cycle, and of a slow rhythm with the period of the respiratory cycle. The autocorrelograms of the discharges of units B and C illustrate that the 8–12 cps periodicity can appear in combination with the cardiac-related and/or the respiratory-related rhythms. These observations rule out the possibility that each of the three common periodicities in whole nerve discharge is mediated by a distinct set of preganglionic sympathetic neurons. Instead, the individual preganglionic sympathetic neuron receives converging inputs from all three central oscillating circuits.

One of the most interesting features of the preganglionic sympathetic neuron is that it behaves probabilistically. That is, statistical techniques are required to demonstrate that the discharges of individual units contain the periodic components that are obvious to the eye in recordings made from whole sympathetic nerve bundles (Gebber and McCall, 1976; Mannard and Polosa, 1973; Seller, 1973). Figure 8 illustrates this point. Preganglionic sympathetic neurons characteristically exhibit low, resting discharge rates (2 impulses per second or lower) in cats with intact neuraxes (see oscillographic traces for units A, B, and C in Fig. 8). These neurons miss firing in a significant number of cardiac cycles. Yet, time interval or autocorrelation analysis reveals that the probability of discharge for about two-thirds of the preganglionic sympathetic units tested is related to the phases of the cardiac cycle (presumably via baroreceptor phasing mechanisms). The post-R wave time-interval his-

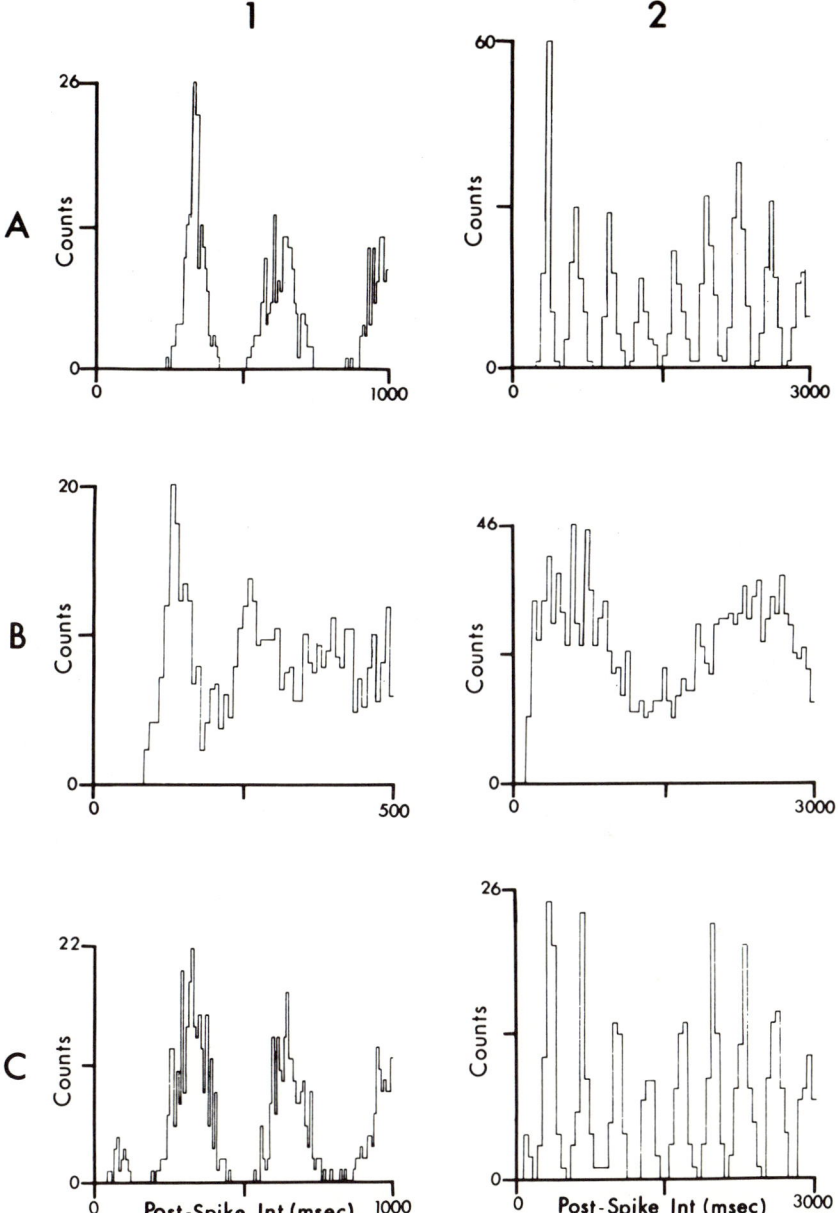

Fig. 7. Autocorrelograms of the discharges of three different preganglionic, cervical sympathetic fibers (A–C). Number of spikes (counts) is plotted against the interval following the spikes that triggered the analysis (at time 0). Trigger spikes are not included in the histograms. Autocorrelograms for each unit are presented on two different times bases (1 and 2). Address bin was 8 msec for histograms in (1) and 48 msec for those in (2). Number of computer sweeps was 371 (A1), 174 (A2), 314 (B1), 125 (B2), 400 (C1) and 100 (C2).

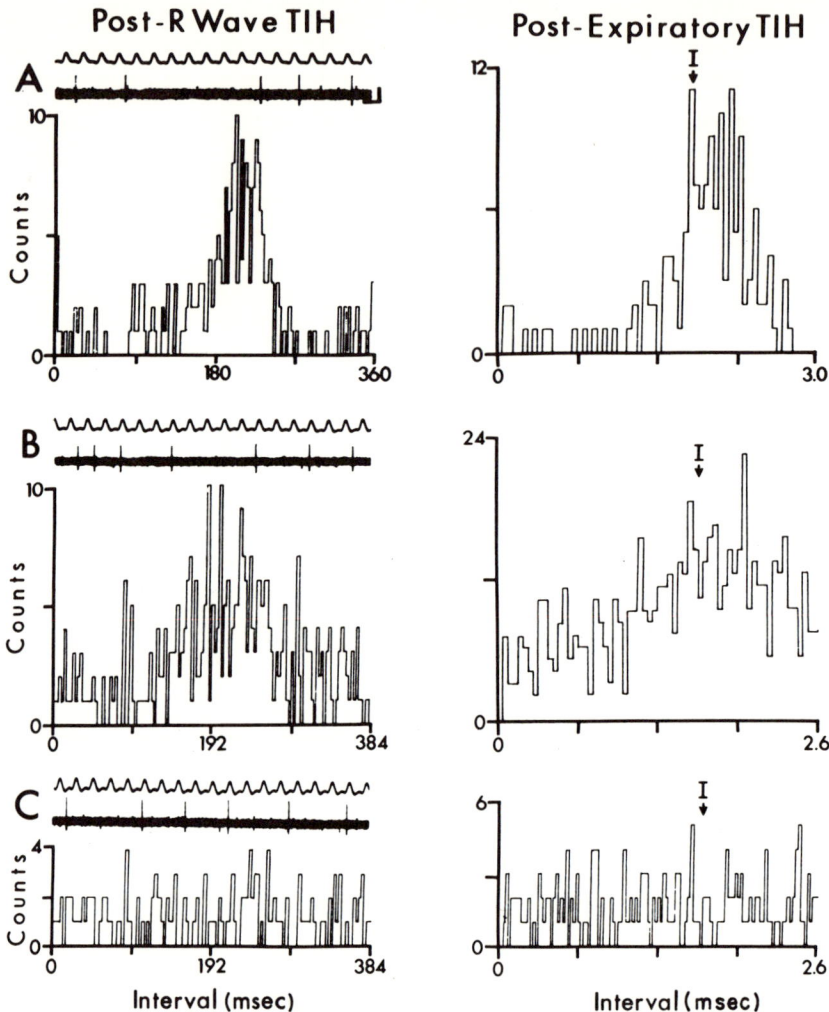

Fig. 8. Patterns of R wave and respiratory-related activity of three preganglionic, cervical sympathetic fibers (A–C) in the vagotomized cat. Units B and C are from the same experiment. Number of spike occurrences (counts) is plotted against the interval following the R wave (*left*) and the start of expiration (*right*) in the time interval histograms (TIH). The abscissa approximates the period of one cardiac cycle in the post-R wave TIH and that of one respiratory cycle in the post-expiratory TIH. The I in post-expiratory TIH denotes the start of inspiration. Post-R wave TIH: address bin was 2.8 msec in A and 3.0 msec in B and C. Number of computer sweeps was 500. Post-expiratory TIH: address bin was 48 msec in A and 40 msec in B and C. Number of computer sweeps was 100. Oscillographic traces above post-R wave TIH show femoral arterial pulse and unitary discharges. Vertical calibration for records of unitary discharge is 200 μV. Horizontal calibration is 360 msec.

tograms in Fig. 8 were constructed from data collected in 500 consecutive cardiac cycles. Note that the probability of discharge of units A and B was greatest approximately 190 msec after the R wave in each cardiac cycle. The respiratory-related periodicity in the discharge of individual preganglionic sympathetic neurons is also most clearly shown with time interval (Fig. 8) or autocorrelation (Fig. 7) analysis. These observations illustrate two important principles of central sympathetic function. First, only a small and continuously changing segment of the total number of preganglionic fibers in a nerve bundle is active at any given time. Thus, tremendous reserve has been built into the system. Second, because preganglionic sympathetic neurons whose discharges are statistically related in time to the R wave of the ECG fail to fire in many cardiac cycles, we are given a clue to the functional significance of synchronization of the activity of populations of brain stem neurons. Synchronization of driving inputs from the brain stem is apparently necessary to bring the preganglionic sympathetic neuron to discharge threshold. We can assume that the number of active inputs and the degree to which they are synchronized are insufficient in those cardiac cycles where the preganglionic neuron fails to fire. The same principle can be applied to the *raison d'être* for those central oscillating circuits responsible for the 8–12 cps and the respiratory-related periodicities in sympathetic nerve discharge.

E.   Inhibitory Interaction between Preganglionic Sympathetic Neurons

We have entertained the question as to whether or not elements of the final common pathway (i.e., preganglionic sympathetic neurons) interact directly with each other (Gebber and Barman, 1979). The results of our study indicate that myelinated preganglionic sympathetic neurons are inhibited by their unmyelinated counterparts. Our experiments were performed on single preganglionic sympathetic neurons located in the T_1–T_3 segments of the cat spinal cord. These neurons were antidromically identified by electrically activating their axons in the cervical sympathetic nerve. Shocks applied to the cervical sympathetic nerve might also excite afferents. To avoid the complication of reflex-induced changes in preganglionic sympathetic neuronal excitability, these afferents were decentralized by extirpation of the T_1–T_3 dorsal root ganglia and by section of the thoracic sympathetic chain, between the T_3 and T_4 white rami. Dorsal root ganglionectomy not only decentralized cervical sympathetic-nerve afferents, which enter the spinal cord over the dorsal roots, but also ventral root afferents (Coggeshall and Ito, 1977; Emery *et al.*, 1977), which arise from dorsal root ganglion cells.

The possibility that preganglionic sympathetic neurons receive inhibition from their neighbors was tested with paired antidromic shocks applied to their axons in the cervical sympathetic nerve. Specifically, the effect of varying the intensity of the conditioning shock was studied on the onset latency and the shape of the antidromic spike produced by the test shock. Trace A in Fig. 9 shows the normalized average of 16 unconditioned, test antidromic responses of a single myelinated, (axonal conduction velocity >2 m/sec) preganglionic sympathetic neuron, on an

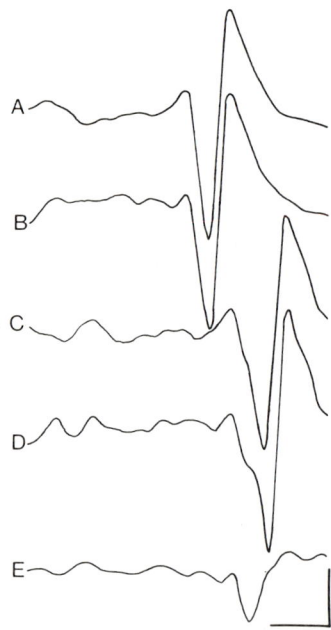

Fig. 9. Changes in test antidromic response of a myelinated, preganglionic sympathetic neuron (axonal conduction velocity, 3.2 m/sec) produced by conditioning shocks of varying intensity. The conditioning and test stimuli were applied to the cervical sympathetic nerve. Traces are normalized averages (16 trials) and show only test response (negativity recorded downward) on an expanded time base. (A) Unconditioned test response. Onset latency was 25 msec. (B) Test response conditioned with a shock (4.8 V) just below threshold for antidromic activation of the unit. Conditioning-test interval was 20 msec in this and subsequent traces. (C) Test response conditioned with shock (5 V) at threshold for antidromic activation of the unit. (D,E) Test responses conditioned with suprathreshold shocks. Intensity of conditioning shock was 12 V in D and 15 V in E. Vertical calibration is 75 μV. Horizontal calibration is 2 msec. Address bin was 100 μsec.

expanded time base. This response was unchanged in onset and shape when conditioned with a shock that was just below the threshold for antidromic activation of the preganglionic sympathetic neuron (Fig. 9B). The interval between the conditioning and the test shocks was 20 msec, in this experiment. As shown in Fig. 9C, the onset of the test antidromic response was delayed approximately 2 msec when conditioned with a stimulus that was at threshold for excitation of the unit under study. Moreover, fractionation of the test response into its initial segment (IS) and somadendritic (SD) components occurred as indicated by the inflection in the rising phase of the spike (negativity recorded downward). Most significantly, the SD, but not the IS spike, was further delayed (trace D) and then blocked (trace E) when the conditioning stimulus was raised from threshold intensity to suprathreshold intensity. Note the accentuated IS–SD break in trace D and the presence of only the IS spike in trace E. These results were obtained in approximately one-third of the myelinated, preganglionic sympathetic neurons studied, and we have interpreted them in the following manner.

The observation that subthreshold conditioning antidromic shocks failed to change the test spike argues against an inhibitory interaction between myelinated, preganglionic sympathetic neurons whose axons have similar thresholds of electrical activation. Thus, barring the existence of autorecurrent inhibition, it seems most likely that changes in the onset and contour of the test response, produced by conditioning shocks that were at threshold for antidromic activation of the preganglionic sympathetic neuron, can be explained by recovery processes intrinsic to the neuron. Delay of the IS spike would arise from slowed conduction velocity due to relative refractoriness of the axon produced by the preceding conditioning response. Fractionation of the test response into its IS and SD components would result from an additional recovery process in the SD region. Further delay or block of the SD spike, produced by raising the intensity of the conditioning shock, however, must be attributed to an inhibitory process of extrinsic origin. Thus, we have concluded that some preganglionic sympathetic neurons whose axons are myelinated receive inhibition from neighboring preganglionic sympathetic neurons whose axons have a considerably higher threshold of electrical activation.

Additional experimentation revealed that intensities of cervical sympathetic nerve stimulation, which blocked the test responses of myelinated, preganglionic sympathetic neurons in our experiments with paired shocks, recruited unmyelinated preganglionic sympathetic neurons (axonal conduction velocity <2m/sec) into the field of antidromic activation. One such experiment is illustrated in Fig. 10. Importantly, the

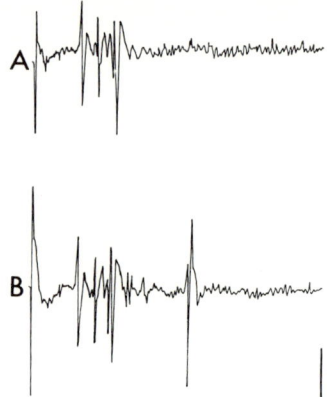

Fig. 10. Multiunit recording from intermediolateral nucleus. Traces are normal-ized averages (32 trials) of antidromic responses of preganglionic sympathetic neurons elicited by single shocks applied once every 2 sec to cervical sympathetic nerve. In-tensity of shock was 7 V in A and 15 V in B. Note that the high intensity shock in B recruited an unmyelinated, preganglionic sympathetic neuron (large spike in cen-ter) into the field of antidromic activation. Axonal conduction velocity of this unit was 1.4 m/sec. Vertical calibration is 75 μV. Horizontal calibration is 20 msec. Address bin was 100 μsec.

onset latencies of antidromic activation of unmyelinated, preganglionic sympathetic neurons were similar to those of the conditioned- test responses of myelinated, preganglionic sympathetic neurons in the paired shock experiments. Therefore, it is possible, on a mathematical basis, to relate the inhibition of myelinated, preganglionic sympathetic neurons to the discharge of their unmyelinated counterparts.

Further studies are needed to elucidate the functional significance of the inhibitory interaction between myelinated and unmyelinated, pre--ganglionic sympathetic neurons. As in other studies, (Fernandez De Molina *et al.,* 1965; Mannard *et al.,* 1977; Polosa, 1967, 1968) inhibitory interactions between myelinated, preganglionic sympathetic neurons could not be demonstrated. Consequently, it seems unlikely that inhibition of myelinated, preganglionic sympathetic neurons by their unmyelinated counterparts forms part of a general negative feedback loop. It appears that the inhibition is lateral rather than recurrent in nature.

It is possible that lateral inhibition involves an interaction between preganglionic sympathetic neurons of vasoconstrictor pathways and cholinergic vasodilator pathways to skeletal muscle. In this regard, vaso-constrictor responses are known to be mediated over pathways containing myelinated, preganglionic sympathetic neurons (Eccles and Wallis, 1976), while Folkow *et al.* (1958) have presented evidence that preganglionic axons in the sympathetic, cholinergic vasodilator pathway are most likely unmyelinated (i.e., C fiber class). Interestingly, it has been established that activation of the sympathetic cholinergic vasodilator system, by stimulation of the hypothalamic defense region, is accompanied by inhibition of vasoconstrictor tone specifically in skeletal muscle (Eliasson *et al.*, 1951; Horeyseck *et al.*, 1976). Whether or not lateral inhibition of myelinated, preganglionic sympathetic neurons by their unmyelinated neighbors accounts for the opposite effects on vasoconstrictor and cholinergic vasodilator outflow to skeletal muscle, produced when the hypothalamus is stimulated, is a question deserving further attention.

It can be assumed that not all unmyelinated, preganglionic sympathetic neurons are components of the cholinergic vasodilator pathway to skeletal muscle, on the basis of the work of Skok *et al.* (1966). They demonstrated that individual neurons in the cat superior cervical ganglion receive converging inputs from unmyelinated and myelinated, preganglionic sympathetic fibers. Thus, it is also possible that lateral inhibition of myelinated, preganglionic sympathetic neurons by their unmyelinated counterparts is indicative of an interaction between sympathoexcitatory neurons subserving identical function (e.g., components of vasoconstrictor pathways). The physiological significance of such an interaction might be related to genesis of the spinal 8–12 cps sympathetic rhythm. Another possibility is that the inhibitory interaction is important in shifting blood flow between different vascular beds (e.g., skin and muscle). In this case, the interaction presumably would occur between myelinated and unmyelinated, preganglionic sympathetic neurons which innervate two separate groups of vasoconstrictor postganglionic cells.

F. Spinal Interneurons in Sympathetic Pathways

Preganglionic sympathetic neurons receive inputs from the brain and periphery, at least in part, over pathways which contain spinal interneurons (Kirchner *et al.*, 1975; Petras and Cummings, 1972). Until recently, however, little information was available concerning the types and locations of spinal interneurons in sympathetic pathways. Regarding this problem, we were interested in answering three specific questions. First, is an interneuron interposed between the terminals of sympathoexcitatory reticulospinal fibers and the preganglionic sympathetic neuron? Second, which element in the sympathoexcitatory pathway (preganglionic neuron or antecedent interneuron) receives bulbospinal inhibition of baroreceptor reflex origin? Third, does the bulbospinal inhibitory pathway contain a spinal interneuron?

Preganglionic sympathetic neurons in the intermediolateral spinal nucleus can be easily identified by backfiring their axons (i.e., by antidromic activation) in peripheral nerve bundles. The problem of identification of interneurons in sympathetic pathways is much more difficult. We approached this problem in the following manner. First, using standard extracellular, microelectrode recording techniques in the cat, we explored the upper thoracic intermediolateral and intermediomedial nuclei for neurons whose probability of discharge was related in time to the R wave of the ECG. Such cells were considered components of sympathetic pathways, in view of their anatomical location in autonomic nuclei and the dependency of their discharge patterns on baroreceptor phasing mechanisms. Second, we determined whether or not units whose discharges were related in time to the R wave could be antidromically activated by stimulation of the cervical or thoracic sympathetic nerves. Those units that were antidromically activated were classified as preganglionic sympathetic neurons. Those units that could not be antidromically activated were classified as interneurons. Finally, we compared the response patterns of preganglionic sympathetic neurons and of nonantidromically activated units to stimuli applied to pressor and depressor sites in the medulla. Such experiments helped to determine whether or not preganglionic neurons and the nonantidromically activated units were closely interconnected components of the same or interacting sympathetic pathways.

The results of our studies in cats (Gebber and McCall, 1976; McCall *et al.*, 1977) are summarized in Fig. 11. The myelinated, preganglionic

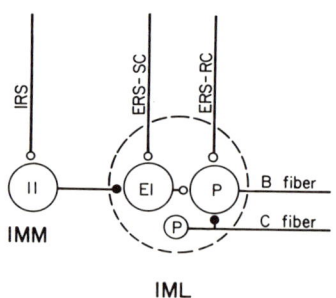

Fig. 11. Summary-wiring diagram of spinal sympathetic network. Unfilled circles are excitatory terminals. Filled circles are inhibitory terminals. EI, spinal interneuron in long latency, sympathoexcitatory pathway; ERS-RC, rapidly conducting reticulospinal fiber in short latency, sympathoexcitatory pathway; ERS-SC, slowly conducting reticulospinal fiber in long latency, sympathoexcitatory pathway; II, spinal interneuron in sympathoinhibitory pathway from baroreceptors; IML, intermediolateral sympathetic spinal nucleus; IMM, intermediomedial sympathetic spinal nucleus; IRS, reticulospinal fiber in sympathoinhibitory pathway from baroreceptors; P-B fiber, myelinated, preganglionic sympathetic neuron; P-C fiber, unmyelinated, preganglionic sympathetic neuron. See text for description of neuronal connections.

sympathetic neuron (P-B fiber) and its antecedent interneuron (EI) have been located in the intermediolateral nucleus (IML). The background discharge patterns of P-B fiber and EI are quite different. The discharges of P-B fiber are characterized by long interspike intervals (of at least 70 msec). In contrast, the EI fires in bursts in which the interspike intervals can be as short as 5 msec. Both unitary types, however, miss firing in many cardiac cycles. The bursting neurons (EI) cannot be antidromically activated by stimulation of preganglionic nerve bundles. Yet, the post-R wave time-interval histograms of the discharges of these neurons are identical to those of antidromically identified P-B fiber. Moreover, EI and P-B fiber are activated with similar onset latencies by single shocks applied to the pressor region of the medulla. These observations led to the conclusion that the nonantidromically activated unit (i.e., EI) is an interneuron, which is interposed between P-B fiber and the terminals of the slowly conducting, sympathoexcitatory reticulospinal fiber (ERS-SC) of the long latency vasopressor pathway (see Section III,B).

Spinal inhibition of baroreceptor reflex origin occurs on EI (see filled circle in Fig. 11) in the sympathoexcitatory pathway. This conclusion was based on the observation that EI exhibited an early phase of inhibition (previously shown, on the basis of whole sympathetic nerve-bundle recordings, to occur at a spinal locus; see Fig. 6) upon electrical stimulation of intramedullary components of the baroreceptor reflex arc, located in the nucleus of the tractus solitarius or the paramedian reticular nucleus. Moreover, it was demonstrated that spinal inhibition of baroreceptor reflex origin is mediated by a spinal interneuron (II) located in the intermediomedial nucleus (IMM). The inhibitory interneuron (II) receives driving inputs from medullospinal projections (IRS) of the baroreceptor reflex arc. This contention is supported by the observations that: (1) discharges from interneuron II were interrupted, within one heartbeat, upon bilateral occlusion of the common carotid arteries of cats whose aortic depressor and vagus nerves were cut; and (2) interneuron II could be activated by single shocks applied to the nucleus of the tractus solitarius (i.e., the medullary nucleus of baroreceptor fiber termination). Importantly, the onset of activation of interneuron II by stimulation of the nucleus of the tractus solitarius was 2 msec shorter than that for the inhibition of EI discharge. This difference is compatible with the idea that the discharge of interneuron II in IMM directly inhibits the EI which is located in IML.

In the past, spinal sympathetic nuclei were believed to function primarily as simple relay stations in pathways from the brain to the periphery. The demonstration that excitatory and inhibitory interneurons exist within these nuclei also indicates that they contain complex integrating circuits. It is possible that the 8–12 cps periodicity in sympathetic nerve discharge (previously shown to be of spinal origin; see Fig. 3) is generated by a spinal interneuronal network. The observation that spinal inhibition occurs on an interneuron rather than directly on the preganglionic sympathetic neuron helps to explain the differential effects exerted by the baroreceptor reflexes on sympathetic nerve discharges produced by stimulation of different brain sites (see Section III,B). Baroreceptor-insensitive sympathetic nerve responses, elicited by stimulation of the hypothalamus and medulla (Gebber *et al.,* 1973; Taylor and Gebber, 1973), presumably project to myelinated preganglionic sympathetic neurons via a pathway which does not include EI. As shown in Fig. 11, the short-latency, baroreceptor-insensitive vasopressor pathway (ERS-RC) may project directly to P-B fiber. Alternatively, other spinal interneuronal types (as of yet unidentified) that do not receive inhibition from the baroreceptor reflexes may be interposed between P-B fiber and the terminals of the rapidly conducting, sympathoexcitatory reticulospinal fiber (ERS-RC). At any rate, it is apparent that the spinal sympathoinhibitory component of the baroreceptor reflexes can be circumvented by selecting the route for excitation of the preganglionic neuron.

The schematic in Fig. 11 also illustrates the inhibitory connection from unmyelinated, preganglionic sympathetic neurons (P-C fiber) to myelinated, preganglionic sympathetic neurons (P-B fiber). As already discussed in Section III,E, the physiological significance of lateral inhibition of P-B fiber by P-C fiber remains to be determined. Furthermore, the driving inputs to P-C fiber are unknown. It is important that future investigations deal with the pathway for lateral inhibition. Does the inhibitory pathway contain an interneuron that functions in a manner analogous to the Renshaw cell in the recurrent inhibitory pathway to alpha motoneurons? In regard to this question, the synaptic activation of neurons in IML by stimulation of preganglionic sympathetic nerves has not been reported. This negative finding, however, does not preclude the existence of a Renshaw-like interneuron in the inhibitory pathway from P-C fiber to P-B fiber in some other spinal sympathetic nucleus.

Inhibition of P-B fiber is mediated over a collateral of P-C fiber in Fig. 11. It should be pointed out, however, that Rethelyi (1972) failed to observe collaterals emanating from the axons of preganglionic sympathetic neurons in the intermediolateral nucleus of the cat spinal cord. Although it would be rash to discount their existence on the basis of the negative findings in one study, the work of Rethelyi and others has provided an alternative pathway for the inhibitory interaction. In many cases, the axon of the preganglionic sympathetic neuron emerges from one of the large dendrites rather than from the soma (Rethelyi, 1972). Moreover, close apposition of dendrites of adjacent preganglionic sympathetic neurons has been reported (Chung *et al.*, 1975; Schramm *et al.*, 1975); and the dendrites of preganglionic sympathetic neurons are capable of propagating action potentials (Fernandez De Molina *et al.*, 1965). Thus, the possibility exists that inhibitory interactions between myelinated and unmyelinated, preganglionic sympathetic neurons are mediated over dendrodendritic connections. It has been previously suggested that dendrodendritic connections are involved in local, recurrent inhibitory circuits within the olfactory bulb and thalamus (Rall and Shepherd, 1968; Shepherd, 1974).

IV. PERSPECTIVE FOR THE FUTURE

A problem that has not yet been effectively treated concerns the identification of brain-stem neurons in sympathetic pathways. Clearly, this problem must be solved, if we are to develop models of those brain-stem oscillating circuits that help generate the background discharges of preganglionic sympathetic nerves and, thus, the neurogenic component of resting blood pressure.

Many neurons in the pontomedullary reticular formation change their discharge rate during drug-induced alterations in blood pressure (see review in Koepchen *et al.*, 1975). Blood-pressure-dependent changes in unitary discharge are most often attributed to baroreceptor reflex effects. The dependency of unitary discharge rate on baroreceptor input, however, is not a valid criterion for the identification of a brain-stem neuron in a sympathetic pathway (i.e., a brain-stem sympathetic neuron). In this regard, it is known that the baroreceptor reflexes influence brain-stem systems that control respiration (Richter and Seller, 1975), somatomotor reflexes (Coote and MacLeod, 1974), and cortical activation (Bonvallet *et al.*, 1954). The same problem arises in the interpretation of studies in which changes in brain-stem unitary discharge have been produced by electrical activation of baroreceptor afferents in the carotid sinus nerve (Koepchen *et al.*, 1975).

As reviewed by Koepchen *et al.* (1975), the brain stem has been explored in the cat, dog, and rabbit for units whose discharges exhibit the cardiac-related rhythm prominent in the activity patterns of afferent baroreceptor and efferent sympathetic nerve bundles. Such neurons have been found in the nucleus of the tractus solitarius but not in the pressor region of the pontomedullary reticular formation. In retrospect, the failure to locate brain-stem reticular neurons whose discharges exhibit a prominent pulse-synchronous component is not surprising, in view of the well-studied firing characteristics of preganglionic sympathetic neurons. As already discussed, these neurons fail to fire in many cardiac cycles. Thus, statistical methods such as post-R wave time-interval analysis and autocorrelation are required to reveal the cardiac-related periodicity in their discharges. Recently, medullary neurons, whose discharges were statistically locked in time to the R wave of the ECG, have been located in the reticular formation by Gebber (1975), Gootman *et al.* (1975), and Stroh-Werz *et al.* (1976). Whether or not these neurons are components of sympathetic pathways, however, remains in question, since (1) unlike the intermediolateral nucleus in the spinal cord, the brain-stem reticular formation is functionally heterogenous in composition; and (2) as already mentioned, the baroreceptor reflexes modulate transmission in a number of reticular networks, in addition to those which subserve sympathetic function. Thus, in my opinion, post-R wave time-interval analysis in functionally heterogenous regions of the brain is not the critical test for identifying components of sympathetic pathways.

Perhaps cross-correlation analysis will provide the definitive test for the identification of brain-stem sympathetic neurons. Cross-correlation is a statistical method that enables one to determine whether two neuronal elements are interconnected synaptically or whether they receive common inputs (Moore *et al.*, 1970). The cross-correlation function between elements A and B is a measure of the expected activity of B relative to the firing times of A. An example of cross-correlation analysis of the whole external carotid, postganglionic sympathetic nerve, and the discharges of a single preganglionic fiber, teased from the cervical sympathetic nerve, is shown in Fig. 12. Unprocessed unitary and whole nerve discharges appear in panel A. The autocorrelograms for the preganglionic unit (panel B) and postganglionic nerve bundle (panel C) show that the discharges of both elements had the same period of oscillation (that of the cardiac cycle). The cross-correlogram (unit→whole nerve) in panel D demonstrates that the periodicities in unitary and whole nerve discharges were locked to each other. Phase lag was essentially zero, in this particular case. It can be concluded from these records that the preganglionic unit was representative of a population of fibers that provided driving inputs to postganglionic neurons of the external carotid, sympathetic nerve.

Recently, Gootman *et al.* (1975) used cross-correlation analysis to demonstrate a relationship between the discharges of a few medullary neurons and those of the whole preganglionic splanchnic sympathetic nerve in the cat. Although preliminary in nature, their experiments may pro-

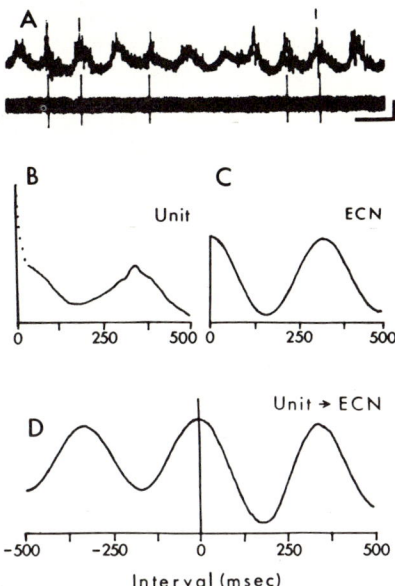

Interval (msec)

Fig. 12. Cross-correlation between discharges of single preganglionic fiber, teased from cervical sympathetic nerve, and those of whole postganglionic external carotid nerve (ECN). (A) Oscillographic traces of ECN (top) and unitary (bottom) discharges. Horizontal calibration is 200 msec. Vertical calibration is 100 μv. (B) Autocorrelogram of unit discharge shows rhythm with period of cardiac cycle. (C) Autocorrelogram of ECN discharge shows same periodicity. (D) Cross-correllogram (unit $\rightarrow$ ECN) shows that periodicities in unitary and ECN discharges are phase-locked. Address bin was 2 msec and number of computer sweeps was 140 for auto- and cross-correlograms.

vide the basis for future studies on the intrinsic organization of brainstem networks responsible for generating background discharges of preganglionic sympathetic neurons.

ACKNOWLEDGMENTS

The research from our laboratory was supported by PHS grant HL13187. Thanks are due to Dr. Susan M. Barman for her critical review of the manuscript.

REFERENCES

Adrian, E. D., Bronk, D. W., and Phillips, G. (1932). Discharges in mammalian sympathetic nerves. *J. Physiol. (London)* **74**, 115–133.

Alexander, R. S. (1946). Tonic and reflex functions of medullary sympathetic cardiovascular centers. *J. Neurophysiol.* **9**, 205–217.

Barman, S. M., and Gebber, G. L. (1976). Basis for synchronization of sympathetic and phrenic nerve discharges. *Am. J. Physiol.* **231,** 1601–1607.

Bernard, C. (1863). "Leçons sur la Physiologie et la Pathologie du Système Nerveux," Vol. 1. Baillière et Fils, Paris.

Bonvallet, M., Dell, P., and Hiebel, G. (1954). Tonus sympathique et activité électrique corticale. *Electroencephalogr. Clin. Neurophysiol.* **6,** 119–144.

Brodal, A. (1957). "The Reticular Formation of the Brain Stem. Anatomical Aspects and Functional Correlations." Oliver & Boyd, London.

Chung, J. M., Chung, K., and Wurster, R. D. (1975). Sympathetic preganglionic neurons of the cat spinal cord: Horseradish peroxidase study. *Brain Res.* **91,** 126–131.

Coggeshall, R. E., and Ito, H. (1977). Sensory fibres in ventral roots L7 and S1 in the cat. *J. Physiol. (London)* **267,** 215–235.

Cohen, M. I., and Gootman, P. M. (1970). Periodicities of efferent discharges of splanchnic nerve of the cat. *Am. J. Physiol.* **218,** 1092–1101.

Coote, J. H., and MacLeod, V. H. (1974). Evidence for the involvement in the baroreceptor reflex of a descending inhibitory pathway. *J. Physiol. (London)* **241,** 477–496.

Dittmar, C. (1873). Uber die Lage des sogenannten Gefasscentrums der Medulla ob longata. *Ber. Verh. K. Saechs. Ges. Wiss., Math.-Phys. Kl.* **25,** 449–479.

Eccles, R., and Wallis, D. I. (1976). Characteristics of the sympathetic innervation of the nictitating membrane and of the vasculature of the nose and tongue of the cat. *J. Neural Trans.* **39,** 113–130.

Eliasson, S., Folkow, B., Lindgren, P., and Uvnäs, B. (1951). Activation of sympathetic vasodilator nerves to the skeletal muscles in the cat by hypothalamic stimulation. *Acta Physiol. Scand.* **23,** 333–351.

Emery, D. G., Ito, H., and Coggeshall, R. E. (1977). Unmyelinated axons in thoracic ventral roots of the cat. *J. Comp. Neurol.* **172,** 37–48.

Fernandez De Molina, A., Kuno, M., and Perl, E. R. (1965). Antidromically-evoked responses from sympathetic preganglionic neurons. *J. Physiol. (London)* **180,** 321–335.

Folkow, B., Johansson, B., and Oberg, B. (1958). The stimulation threshold of different sympathetic fibre groups as correlated to their functional differentiation. *Acta Physiol. Scand.* **44,** 146–156.

Gebber, G. L. (1975). The probabilistic behavior of central "vasomotor" neurons. *Brain Res.* **96,** 142–146.

Gebber, G. L. (1976). Basis for phase relations between baroreceptor and sympathetic nervous discharge. *Am. J. Physiol.* **230,** 263–270.

Gebber, G. L., and Barman, S. M. (1977). Brain stem vasomotor circuits involved in the genesis and entrainment of sympathetic nervous rhythms. *In* "Hypertension and Brain Mechanisms" (W. De Jong, A. P. Provoost, and A. P. Shapiro, eds.), Progress in Brain Research, Vol. 47, pp. 61–75. Elsevier, Amsterdam.

Gebber, G. L., and Barman, S. M. (1979). Inhibitory interaction between preganglionic sympathetic neurons. *In* "Nervous System and Hypertension" (P. Meyer and H. Schmitt, eds.), pp. 137–145. Wiley, New York.

Gebber, G. L., and McCall, R. B. (1976). Identification and discharge patterns of spinal sympathetic interneurons. *Am. J. Physiol.* **231,** 722–733.

Gebber, G. L., Taylor, D. G., and Weaver, L. C. (1973). Electrophysiological studies on organization of central vasopressor pathways. *Am. J. Physiol.* **224,** 470–481.

Gootman, P. M., Cohen, M. I., Piercey, M. P., and Wolotsky, P. (1975). A search for medullary neurons with activity patterns similar to those in sympathetic nerves. *Brain Res.* **87**, 395–406.

Green, J. H., and Heffron, P. F. (1967). Observations on the origin and genesis of a rapid sympathetic rhythm. *Arch. Int. Pharmacodyn. Ther.* **169**, 403–411.

Heymans, C., and Neil, E. (1958). "Reflexogenic Areas of the Cardiovascular System." Little, Brown, Boston, Massachusetts.

Horeyseck, G., Jänig, W., Kirchner, F., and Thämer, V. (1976). Activation and inhibition of muscle and cutaneous postganglionic neurones to hindlimb during hypothalamically induced vasoconstriction and atropine-sensitive vasodilation. *Pfluegers Arch.* **34**, 231–240.

Kirchner, F., Wyszogrodski, I., and Polosa, C. (1975). Some properties of sympathetic neuron inhibition by depressor area and intraspinal stimulation. *Pfluegers Arch.* **357**, 349–360.

Koepchen, H. P., Langhorst, P., and Seller, H. (1975). The problem of identification of autonomic neurons in the lower brain stem. *Brain Res.* **87**, 375–393.

Koizumi, K., Seller, H., Kaufman, A., and Brooks, C. McC. (1971). Pattern of sympathetic discharges and their relation to baroreceptor and respiratory activities. *Brain Res.* **27**, 281–294.

Loewy, A. D., and Burton, H. (1977). Efferent projections from nuclei of the solitary tract in the cat. *Soc. Neurosci. Abstr.* **3**, 71.

McCall, R. B., and Gebber, G. L. (1975). Brain stem and spinal synchronization of sympathetic nervous discharge. *Brain Res.* **88**, 139–143.

McCall, R. B., Gebber, G. L., and Barman, S. M. (1977). Spinal interneurons in the baroreceptor reflex arc. *Am. J. Physiol.* **232**, H657–H665.

Mannard, A., and Polosa, C. (1973). Analysis of background firing of single sympathetic preganglionic neurons of the cat cervical nerve. *J. Neurophysiol.* **36**, 398–408.

Mannard, A., Rajchgot, P., and Polosa, C. (1977). Effect of post-impulse depression on background firing of sympathetic preganglionic neurons. *Brain Res.* **126**, 243–261.

Miura, M., and Reis, D. J. (1969). Termination and secondary projections of carotid sinus nerve in the cat brain stem. *Am. J. Physiol.* **217**, 142–153.

Moore, G. P., Segundo, J. P., Perkel, D. H., and Levitan, H. (1970). Statistical signs of synaptic interaction in neurons. *Biophys. J.* **10**, 876–900.

Owsjannikow, P. (1871). Die tonischen und reflectorischen Centren der Gefassnerven. *Ber. Verh. K. Saechs. Ges. Wiss., Math.-Phys. Kl.* **23**, 135–147.

Palkovits, M., and Zaborsky, L. (1977). Neuroanatomy of central cardiovascular control. Nucleus tractus solitarii: Afferent and efferent neuronal connections in relation to the baroreceptor reflex arc. *In* "Hypertension and Brain Mechanisms" (W. De Jong, A. P. Provoost, and A. P. Shapiro, eds.), Progress in Brain Research, Vol. 47, pp. 9–34. Elsevier, Amsterdam.

Peiss, C. N. (1965). Concepts of cardiovascular regulation: Past, present and future. *In* "Nervous Control of the Heart" (W. C. Randall, ed.), pp. 154–197. Williams & Wilkins, Baltimore, Maryland.

Petras, J. M., and Cummings, J. F. (1972). Autonomic neurons in the spinal cord of the rhesus monkey: A correlation of the fiindings of cytoarchitectonics and sympathectomy with fiber degeneration following dorsal rhizotomy. *J. Comp. Neurol.* **146**, 189–218.

Polosa, C. (1967). The silent period of sympathetic preganglionic neurons. *Can. J. Physiol. Pharmacol.* **45**, 1033–1045.

Polosa, C. (1968). Spontaneous activity of sympathetic preganglionic neurons. *Can. J. Physiol. Pharmacol.* **46**, 887–896.

Rall, W., and Shepherd, G. M. (1968). Theoretical reconstruction of field potentials and dendrodendritic synaptic interactions in olfactory bulb. *J. Neurophysiol.* **31**, 884–915.

Ranson, S. W., and Billingsley, P. R. (1916). Vasomotor reactions from stimulation of the floor of the fourth ventricle. *Am. J. Physiol.* **41**, 85–90.

Rethelyi, M. (1972). Cell and neuropil architecture of the intermediolateral (sympathetic) nucleus of cat spinal cord. *Brain Res.* **46**, 203–213.

Ricardo, J. A., and Koh, E. T. (1977). Direct projections from the nucleus of the solitary tract to the hypothalamus, amygdala and other forebrain structures in the rat. *Anat. Rec.* **187**, 693.

Richter, D. W., and Seller, H. (1975). Baroreceptor effects on medullary respiratory neurones of the cat. *Brain Res.* **86**, 168–171.

Scheibel, M. E., and Schiebel, A. B. (1958). Structural substrates for integrative patterns in the brainstem reticular core. *In* "Reticular Formation of the Brain" (H. H. Jasper, L. D. Proctor, R. S. Knighton, W. C. Noshay and R. T. Costello, eds.), pp. 31–55. Little, Brown, Boston, Massachusetts.

Schramm, L. P., Adair, J. R., Stribling, J. M., and Gray, L. P. (1975). Preganglionic innervation of the adrenal gland of the rat: a study using horseradish peroxidase. *Exp. Neurol.* **49**, 540–553.

Seller, H. (1973). The discharge pattern of single units in thoracic and lumbar white rami in relation to cardiovascular events. *Pfluegers Arch.* **343**, 317–330.

Seller, H., and Illert, M. (1969). The localization of the first synapse in the carotid sinus baroreceptor reflex pathway and its alteration of the afferent input. *Pfluegers Arch.* **306**, 1–19.

Shepherd, G. M. (1974). "The Synaptic Organization of the Brain." Oxford Univ. Press, London and New York.

Skok, V. I., Ivanov, A. Y., and Buklova, R. P. (1966). Convergence in cat superior cervical ganglion. *Fiziol. Zh. (Kiev)* **12**, 721–727.

Snyder, D. W., and Gebber, G. L. (1973). Relationships between medullary depressor region and central vasopressor pathways. *Am. J. Physiol.* **225**, 1129–1137.

Spyer, K. M. (1972). Baroreceptor sensitive neurones in the anterior hypothalamus of the cat. *J. Physiol. (London)* **224**, 245–257.

Stroh-Werz, M., Langhorst, P., and Camerer, H. (1976). Neuronal activity with relation to cardiac rhythm in the lower brain stem of the dog. *Brain Res.* **106**, 293–305.

Taylor, D. G., and Gebber, G. L. (1973). Sympathetic unit responses to stimulation of cat medulla. *Am. J. Physiol.* **225**, 1138–1146.

Taylor, D. G., and Gebber, G. L. (1975). Baroreceptor mechanisms controlling sympathetic nervous rhythms of central origin. *Am. J. Physiol.* **228**, 1002–1013.

Thomas, M. R., and Calaresu, F. R. (1972). Responses of single units in the medial hypothalamus to electrical stimulation of the carotid sinus nerve in the cat. *Brain Res.* **44**, 49–62.

Wang, S. C., and Ranson, S. W. (1939a). Autonomic responses to electrical stimulation of the lower brain stem. *J. Comp. Neurol.* **71**, 437–455.

Wang, S. C., and Ranson, S. W. (1939b). Descending pathways from hypothalamus to the medulla and spinal cord. Observations on blood pressure and bladder responses. *J. Comp. Neurol.* **71**, 457–472.

4

The Nucleus Tractus
Solitarii (NTS) and
Experimental
Neurogenic
Hypertension

Donald J. Reis

NEURAL CONTROL OF CIRCULATION

I. THE BRAIN AND HYPERTENSION

The cause of essential hypertension remains obscure (Pickering, 1968; Laragh, 1974; Genest *et al.*, 1977). In the past, the search for an etiology has focused on either the pathogenetic role of the kidneys, body fluids, and electrolytes, or a defective regulation of the aldosterone-renin/angiotensin system. In recent years, however, an increased awareness has developed that the central nervous system (CNS) may play an important role in the expression of the disease (Chalmers, 1975; De Jong *et al.*, 1977; De Quattro and Miura, 1973; Dickenson, 1965; Julius and Esler, 1976; Onesti *et al.*, 1976; Reis and Doba, 1974; Zanchetti, 1972). The question may even be raised as to whether or not the CNS itself may be the site of the primary defect.

Support for the theory that the CNS has a role in the expression of hypertension has evolved from several parallel lines of evidence. First, the development of new and sensitive methods for the detection of circulating catecholamines has indicated that there is a population of patients with hypertension in which the levels of circulating catecholamines are elevated (De Quattro and Miura, 1973; Koch-Weser, 1973; Louis *et al.*, 1973; Mendlowitz and Vlachakis, 1976). Second, it is a fact that many drugs, effective in the treatment of the human disease, block sympathetic neurotransmission; several of these drugs, including α-methyldopa and clonidine, act through central mechanisms (De Jong and Nijkamp, 1975, 1976; De Jong *et al.*, 1975; Finch *et al.*, 1975; Haeusler, 1974; Helse and Kroneberg, 1973; Henning and Robinson, 1971; Kobinger and Walland, 1972a,b; Korner *et al.*, 1974; Louis *et al.*, 1973; Nijkamp and De Jong, 1975; Srivastava *et al.*, 1973). Finally, the introduction of 24-hour recordings of arterial pressure from indwelling arterial catheters has given further support to the view that at least some patients with hypertension demonstrate an increased variability of their arterial pressure (lability) and exaggerated responses of arterial pressure to behavioral and environmental stimuli (exaggerated reactivity) (Littler *et al.*, 1972, 1976). This latter feature may in fact be the link between life stress, the brain, emotionality, and hypertension.

A. Relationship of Sympathetic Nervous System to Blood Vessel Pathology

The precise relationship between the augmented sympathetic nerve activity and hypertensive disease still remains to be elucidated. One popular hypothesis, that of Folkow (Sivertsson, 1970; Folkow, 1971), has suggested that augmented sympathetic nervous activity, even intermittent and possibly guided by heightened states of vigilance or emotionality (Folkow and Rubenstein, 1966; Lamprecht *et al.*, 1973; Reis and Doba, 1974), can, *when sustained,* lead to structural or biochemical changes in the blood vessel wall. These changes, consisting of vascular hyperplasia, result in a reduction of the wall–lumen ratio and a long-lasting increase in vascular resistance, which ultimately becomes independent of the initiating neural stimulus. Such a transmutation of a transient to an established state of heightened vascular resistance might serve to link the labile and fixed forms of neurogenic hypertension. It has been demonstrated that increased sympathetic neural activity, even if brief, can lead to prolonged changes in cyclic nucleotide metabolism in the vessel wall of rats, comparable to those produced in other forms of experimental or spontaneous hypertension in that species (Amer *et al.*, 1974, 1975).

B. Brain Stem and Control of Circulation

For any link between the sympathetic nervous system and hypertension, we must consider the CNS as the potential site for disordered neural function. It has long been recognized that the CNS is essential for modulating the background discharge of sympathetic neurons, essential for maintaining vasomotor tone and, thereby, the tonic level of sympathetic discharge (Alexander, 1946; Kumada *et al.*, 1979). It is also essential, in response to more general homeostatic drives, for processing reflex and behavioral (phasic) inputs to the sympathetic outflow, and redistributing organ blood flow in a manner appropriately organized to meet the local metabolic requirements during behavior.

While phasic control of the sympathetic nervous system appears integrated at virtually every segment of the neuraxis, the tonic control of vasomotor background appears to depend largely on the integrity of the medulla oblongata (Alexander, 1946; Kumada *et al.*, 1979). Experiments dating back to the middle of the last century have demonstrated that the removal of structures rostral to the pontomedullary junction fail to reduce arterial pressure in anesthetized animals. Progressive transections of the brain stem below this segment, however, result in a progressive decline in blood pressure until a minimal value is reached with lesions somewhere close to the C1 level. Such evidence has led to the concept that neurons intrinsic to the medulla oblongata serve as "tonic vasomotor centers" whose integrity is necessary for normal maintenance of arterial pressure.

Recently, we have identified a highly localized region of the medulla which lies in the dorsal tegmentum and includes portions of the parvocellular and gigantocellular reticular nuclei (Dampney *et al.*, 1979; Kumada *et al.*, 1979) (Fig. 1). This area serves as a receptor for initiation of the hypertension produced by brain stem ischemia or distortion. Lesions restricted to this area result in a fall of arterial pressure comparable to that produced by spinal section. We have proposed that this region represents the tonic vasomotor center of the brain stem (Dampney *et al.*, 1979; Kumada *et al.*, 1979).

The organization of the medullary vasomotor areas is complex. Electrical stimulation has demonstrated that the lower brain stem can be divided into regions from which a rise of arterial pressure can be elicited (the so-called vasopressor centers) and regions from which electrical stimulation will reduce the arterial pressure by inhibition of sympathetic discharge (the so-called vasodepressor centers) (Alexander, 1946). Under normal circumstances the tonic level of arterial pressure is maintained.

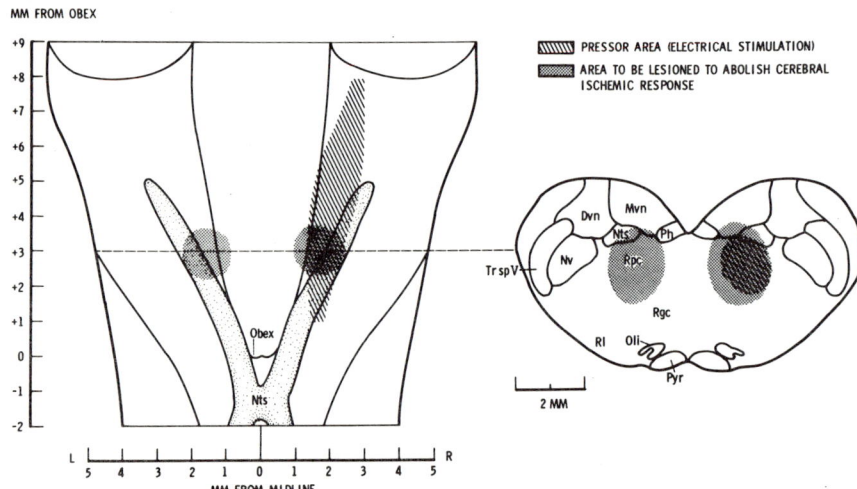

Fig. 1. Localization of tonic vasomotor center in rabbit brain. Left: Dorsal view of floor of fourth ventricle. Right: Cross section of the medulla corresponding to dotted line. Crosshatched area represents area from which the vasomotor response, identical to the cerebral ischemic response, is elicited by electrical stimulation. Stippled area corresponds to zone which, when lesioned bilaterally, results in a permanent fall of arterial pressure to levels comparable to those produced by spinal transection. Dvn, descending vestibular nucleus; Mvn, medial vestibular nucleus: Nv, nucleus of trigeminal nerve; Nts, nucleus of solitary tract; Oli, nucleus of the inferior olive; Ph, nucleus praepositus hypoglossi; Pyr, pyramidal tract; Rgc, nucleus reticularis gigantocellularis; Rl, nucleus reticularis lateralis; Rpc, nucleus reticularis parvocellularis, TrspV, spinal tract of trigeminal nerve. (From Kumada *et al.*, 1979.)

This indicates that the pressor and depressor systems in life balance each other out, which results in normal levels of arterial pressure.

C. Animal Models of Hypertension with Manipulation of the CNS

Any theory of hypertension involving the CNS must consider the possibility that the hypertension results from imbalances in the counterpoised pressor and depressor systems of the brain stem. Such imbalances must favor either (1) facilitation of pressor centers; or (2) inhibition of the inhibitory centers. Either condition would lead to development of augmented sympathetic discharge, increased peripheral vascular resistance, and finally, arterial hypertension.

Attempts made in the past to produce hypertension by manipulations of the CNS or its reflex systems have not been successful in the production of sustained hypertension (Cowley et al., 1973). The experimental studies have attempted to produce hypertension in two ways: (1) by facilitating sympathetic drive; and (2) by withdrawing inhibition to the sympathetic outflow.

The most common group of studies has been those aimed at directly increasing sympathetic excitation. In general, these have included techniques for chronic electrical stimulation of the brain (Folkow and Rubenstein, 1966), by rendering the brain chronically ischemic (Dickenson, 1965), by submitting animals to chronic emotional stress, or by classical conditioning (Farris et al., 1945; Folkow and Rubenstein, 1966; Henry et al., 1971; Herd et al., 1969; Lamprecht et al., 1973).

In general, attempts to produce chronic hypertension by excitation of sympathetic discharge have not resulted in sustained hypertension. Hypertension has primarily been produced during the period of stimulation, and blood pressure gradually returns to or toward normal after stimulation has terminated. The permanence of such hypertension has been, at best, questionable.

Attempts to produce hypertension by withdrawal of inhibitory inputs to sympathetic neurons have been less common. Until recently, almost all such studies have attempted to reduce sympathetic inhibition by interruption of arterial baroreceptors, i.e., sinoaortic denervation (see Reis and Doba, 1974). Such studies have been conducted in rats, cats, dogs, and rabbits. The question has been raised recently as to whether or not the changes in arterial pressure produced by sinoaortic denervation is permanent. The primary challenge is that sinoaortic denervation produces lability and exaggerated reactivity of the arterial pressure rather than fixed hypertension (Cowley et al., 1973). If care is not taken to study animals under strict behavioral control, the exaggerated reactivity may lead to the false impression that elevated arterial pressure is fixed.

In summary, attempts to produce a model in animals that have comparable features to essential hypertension in man have not been successful by techniques aimed at increasing sympathetic discharge by behavioral or environmental manipulation, nor by withdrawing inhibition of sympathetic nerves by sinoaortic denervation. The models have failed to produce a tonically sustained elevation of arterial pressure.

D. Objectives and Goals of Animal Models of Neurogenic Hypertension

It is evident that the promotion of a hypothesis identifying the CNS as a site of causality of hypertension in animals requires that it be demonstrated that: (1) the imbalances within the brain, either structural or biochemical, can lead to hypertension; (2) the hypertension is neurogenic; (3) the hypertension is sustained; (4) the hypertension is the principal physiological abnormality and is not associated with changes in behavior; and (5) the hypertension leads to characteristic cardiovascular pathology. Desirable in such models would be the expression of other features sometimes linked with the disease, including the lability and exaggerated reactivity of the arterial pressure.

It should be emphasized that such a model will not *prove* the etiology of essential hypertension in man. Rather, it will only demonstrate that an impairment of the CNS can *potentially* produce a vascular disorder comparable, in many of its aspects, to the disease.

II. NTS HYPERTENSION

Over the past several years, our laboratory has pursued a new approach for the production of hypertension by manipulation of the CNS (Cowley *et al.*, 1973; Doba and Reis, 1973, 1974; Farris *et al.*, 1945; Nathan and Reis, 1977; Nathan *et al.*, 1978; Reis *et al.*, 1979; Snyder *et al.*, 1978a,b). The strategy has been to impair the function of inhibitory centers of the lower brain stem, specifically those integrating baroreceptor reflexes. By destruction of the central site of integration of baroreceptor activity in the brain, the NTS, we have been able to produce a model of hypertension in animals that appears to be sustained. We have also investigated the consequences of impairing a specific catecholaminergic input into the NTS to determine if a neurochemical abnormality in the brain stem can lead to aberrant regulation of cardio-vascular control. These studies will be reviewed.

A.   The NTS and Blood Pressure Control

A renewal of interest in the central mechanisms mediating baroreflexes began in the early 1960's (Hilton, 1963; Reis and Cuenod, 1964) with observations that baroreceptor reflex responses were under both tonic and phasic control of regions of the brain remote from the primary site of integration. At the time of these discoveries, it was not known where arterial baroreceptor afferents terminated in the brain, although it was supposed that they probably projected into the primary afferent column of the medulla, the NTS. In the 1960s and 1970s, several investigators unequivocally demonstrated, by use of traditional anatomical and elec-trophysiological techniques, that a primary site of termination of baro-receptor afferents was in the NTS, or specifically, in the intermediate portion of the area of the nucleus, lying at about the level of the obex (Cottle, 1964; Chiba and Doba, 1976).

One interesting finding, perhaps the progenitor of the present results, was the observation by Miura and Reis (1972) that, whereas bilateral lesions of the NTS in the anesthetized cat resulted in the disappearance of all reflex activity arising from arterial baro- and chemoreceptors, those animals, nevertheless, failed to develop elevation of their arterial pres-sure. This observation was unexpected since sinoaortic denervation re-sulted in subacute hypertension both in anesthetized and unanesthetized cats (Reis and Cuenod, 1964).

An attempt to establish whether or not the failure to produce hyper-tension by NTS lesions in cats was consequent to an effect of anesthesia led Doba and Reis (1973) to undertake studies in which NTS lesions were placed in rats that were instrumented for recording of their arterial pressure while awake and unanesthetized. The general protocol for these and subsequent studies was to instrument the animals under a short-acting anesthesia (halothane), obtain baseline cardiovascular values upon recovery, reanesthetize the animals and insert brain lesions, and record changes in cardiovascular activity upon discontinuation of the anesthetic.

B.   NTS Hypertension in the Rat

In the rat, bilateral electrolytic lesions of the NTS result in the devel-opment of arterial hypertension within minutes after recovery from anesthesia (Fig. 2). The elevation of systolic pressure, usually greater than 200 mm Hg, is entirely of neurogenic origin and is due to a massive in-

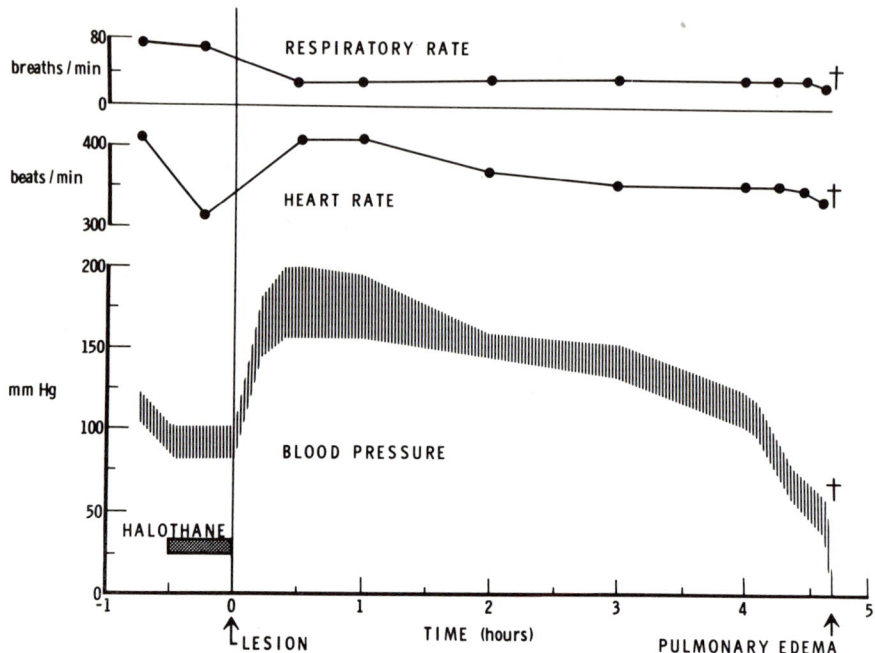

Fig. 2. Time course of changes in systemic arterial blood pressure, heart rate, and respiratory rate in a representative unanesthetized rat after production of bilateral lesions in the NTS. Just prior to death, the rat developed pulmonary edema. (From Doba and Reis, 1973.)

crease in peripheral vasoconstriction consequent to enhanced discharge of preganglionic sympathetic neurons. The vasoconstriction, mediated by α-adrenergic receptors, is regionally differentiated, being most intense in the skin, muscle, and colon (Snyder *et al.*, 1978a). The redistribution of blood flow is similar to that associated with interruption of baroreceptors and different from other forms of arterial hypertension (see Snyder *et al.*, 1978a).

The location of the structures rostral to the midbrain that are essential for the expression of hypertension is unknown. Recent studies by M. J. Brody *et al.* (1979) have suggested that the NTS hypertension can be aborted by small lesions in ventral portions of the anterior third ventricle, possibly identifying this as the rostral site essential for the development of the elevated blood pressure.

The expression of hypertension is dependent on the integrity of descending noradrenergic projections to the spinal cord (Doba and Reis, 1974). The intracisternal administration of the drug 6-hydroxydopamine

(6-OHDA) will block the development of NTS hypertension even when the adrenal glands are intact. On the other hand, ascending noradrenergic (and dopaminergic) projections do not appear to influence NTS hypertension because intrahypothalamic injections of 6-OHDA, producing massive degeneration of ascending catecholaminergic projections (Doba and Reis, 1974), do not influence its development.

These studies established that an imbalance of an inhibitory region of the brain stem of the rat could lead to acute fulminating, neurogenic hypertension. The hypertension itself was so intense that it led to myocardial overload, heart failure, and death. The "fulminating" quality of the hypertension was secondary to vasoconstriction. The mechanism of hypertension was due, presumably, to the destruction of baroreceptor influence centrally, with the release of sympathetic vasomotor neurons from inhibition.

C.   Chronic Labile Hypertension in Cat

The rapid development of malignant heart failure following NTS lesions in rat led us to determine whether or not a larger animal, i.e., a cat, could survive the initial sympathetic overactivity following comparable lesions of the brain (Nathan and Reis, 1977). Within minutes after placement of NTS lesions and termination of anesthesia, the arterial pressure of the cat, as in the rat, begins to rise, reaching an average of 144 mm Hg. However, after an initial phase of hypertension, the pressure drops and reaches normal values 24 hours later. Whereas some animals develop cardiac failure and even die with pulmonary edema, most survive and develop profound and persistent cardiovascular disturbances.

Cats with long-standing bilateral lesions of NTS develop a syndrome characterized by five cardinal features (Nathan and Reis, 1977).

1.   Lability of Arterial Pressure

Cats with NTS lesions exhibit a marked second-to-second variability (lability) of blood pressure which is characterized by marked spontaneous fluctuations with both elevations and depressions often as great as 100 mmHg (Figs. 3 and 4). The lability is influenced by environmental stimulation and is greater during the day in a laboratory environment. The assessment of lability and the capacity to measure the average arterial pressure in the face of fluctuations has been achieved by computer-assisted analysis (Fig. 4) (Cowley et al., 1973; Snyder et al., 1978b). By

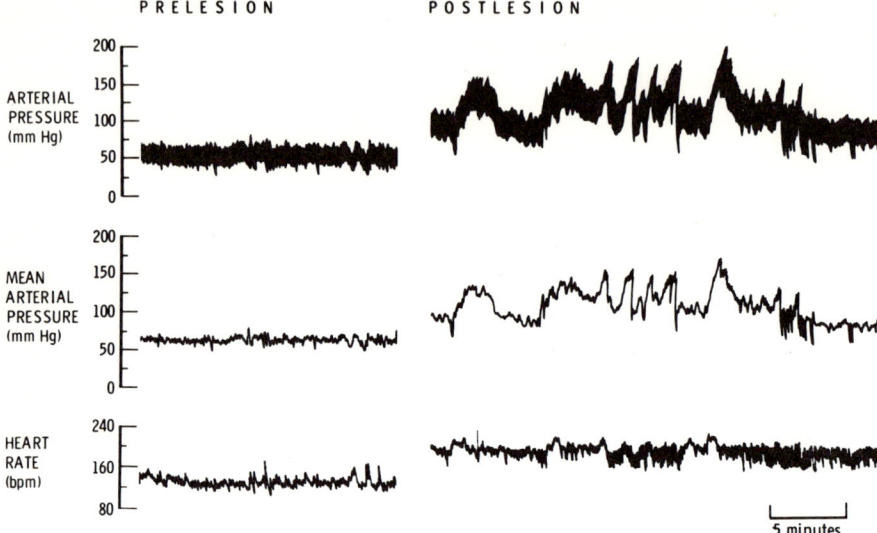

Fig. 3. Labile changes in arterial pressure following NTS lesions in cat. The pre-lesion tracing was taken two days before placement of the lesions, when the cat was in quiet wakefulness and lying down. The postlesion result was obtained one week after placement of lesions during a comparable behavior. Note the extreme lability of the arterial pressure. (From Nathan and Reis, 1977.)

rapidly sampling cardiovascular variables and by the generation of frequency histograms, it has been possible to assess the average level of arterial pressure or heart rate, as well as the lability expressed as the standard deviation of the mean.

2. Sustained Hypertension

The arterial pressure of chronically lesioned animals is significantly elevated above controls. This elevation appears permanent and is dependent upon sympathetic nerves.

3. Exaggerated Responsivity

There is exaggerated responsivity of the arterial pressure during spontaneous or evoked behaviors, or in response to environmental stimulation (Fig. 5).

4. Fixed Tachycardia

The heart rate of lesioned cats is permanently elevated.

5. Absence or Marked Attenuation of Baroreceptor Reflex

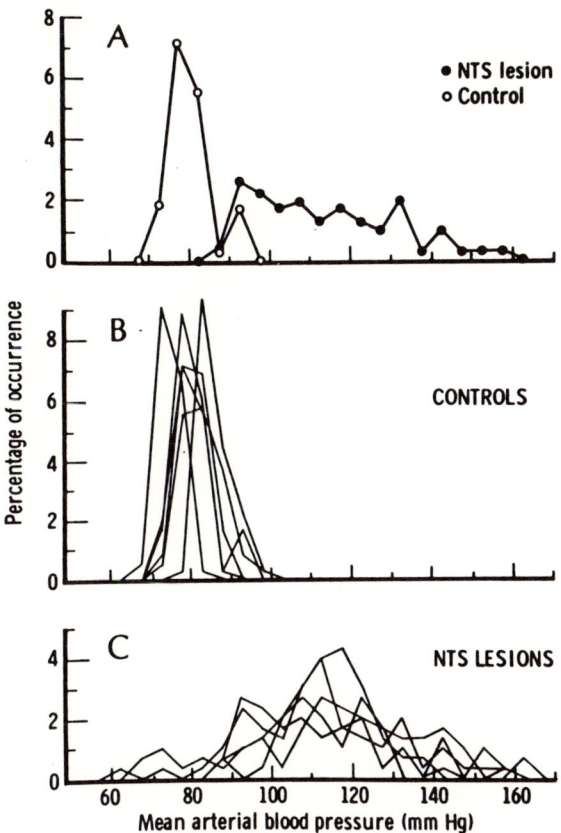

Fig. 4. Daytime frequency histogram of mean arterial pressure in normal and NTS-lesioned cats. (A) individual cat before (O) and one week after (●) placement of the lesions. (B) Overlay of six normal cats 1 week after the sham operation. (C) Overlay of five cats 1 week after placement of NTS lesions. Note the increased lability of the mean arterial pressure in the NTS-lesioned cats. (From Nathan and Reis, 1977.)

D. Enhancement of Conditioned Arterial Pressure Responses after NTS Lesions in Cat

The exaggerated responses of the arterial pressure to environmental stimuli following the placement of bilateral lesions of NTS in cats have suggested that even larger and more sustained elevations might be produced by methods of classical conditioning. Such conditioning procedures, including controlled presentation of sensory stimuli which signal the occurrence of a noxious event, have been used by others to produce

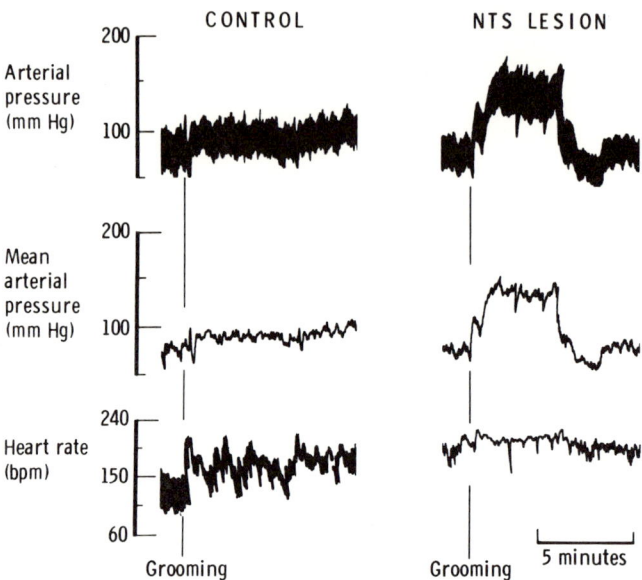

Fig. 5. Facilitation of pressor response to grooming after NTS lesions. (From Nathan and Reis, 1977.)

conditioned elevations in arterial pressure (Harris and Brady, 1974; Reis and Doba, 1974).

Nathan *et al.* (1978) conditioned cats with NTS lesions, comparing them with sham-operated controls. The unconditioned stimulus was an electric shock delivered through an implanted electrode in the flank; the conditioned response was a tone of high frequency; and the con-trolled stimulus was a tone of low frequency. The conditioning proce-dure was conducted for 30 daily sessions. The duration of the tones was gradually lengthened as training progressed so that by sessions 21–30, it was 60 seconds long.

Cats with NTS lesions demonstrated substantially larger conditioned responses of their arterial pressure than did their matched controls (Fig. 6). The rise of arterial pressure occurred at earlier sessions, and by the end of the training period, the rise of arterial pressure was five times greater than that of the controls. Thus, by the end of the trial, the NTS lesion group showed an average increase of 35 mm Hg, in contrast to the 7 mm Hg recorded from the controls ($p<.001$).

The conditioned pressor responses obtained in cats with NTS lesions were substantially larger than those previously produced by classical

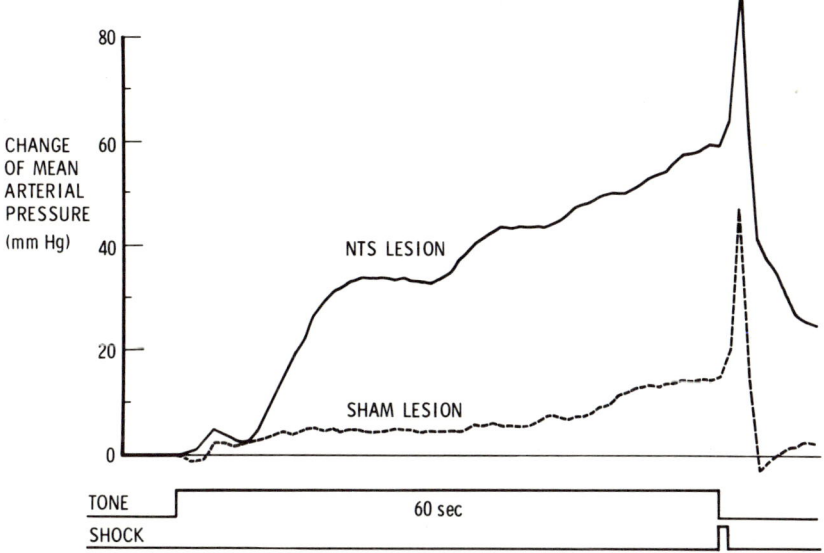

Fig. 6. Conditional increase in arterial pressure in six cats with bilateral electro-lytic lesions of NTS (NTS lesion) and six sham-operated controls. The tracings represent average values of six cats for each group. Resting average arterial pressure did not differ between groups. The tracings at the bottom of the record indicate the duration of a tone and shock. Recordings represent thirtieth trial. Note facilitated pressor response in NTS-lesioned animals. (From Nathan *et al.*, 1978.)

conditioning, and were generally in excess of those obtained by operant conditioning (Harris and Brady, 1974). These findings demonstrate that baroreceptors serve to buffer emotionally elicited pressor responses and, more importantly, that they may counterbalance environmental stimuli, which might lead to exaggeration of the arterial pressure.

The observation that NTS lesions in cat facilitate conditioned elevation of blood pressure leads to a testable hypothesis: For the environment or emotions to produce hypertension, it is essential for baroreflex integration to be impaired. Thus, the failure of stress to produce sustained hypertension in animal models may be explained by the efficacy of baroreceptor mechanisms to offset the emotional drive to sympathetic neurons. However, in a setting of impaired baroreflex function, emotional stress may act to produce disease. Conversely, baroreflex dysfunction alone may also fail to produce hypertension. Only when coupled with environmental or emotional stress will sustained hypertension appear.

E. Implications of Studies of Electrolytic Lesions of NTS
for Understanding Hypertension in Man

The preceding studies in rat and cat have identified the NTS as an important area of the brain stem with respect to the regulation of arterial pressure. Destruction of NTS can lead to abnormalities of arterial pressure with some similarities to the human disease. Thus, in the larger animal, such as the cat, the lesions led to a chronic elevation of arterial pressure without evident changes in the normal behavior of the animal, without lability of arterial pressure, and without exaggerated reactivity of the arterial pressure. These findings have demonstrated, for the first time, that an abnormality of the CNS can lead to chronic hypertension.

In man, lesions of the CNS resulting in hypertension are rare and usually are associated with serious neurological diseases (Reis and Doba, 1974). It is not feasible, therefore, to accept the proposition that essential hypertension is due to bilateral lesions of NTS in the human. A more attractive hypothesis is that chemical imbalances of the brain, possibly involving NTS, may themselves establish conditions leading inexorably to the production of high blood pressure.

III. LABILITY OF ARTERIAL PRESSURE PRODUCED BY IMPAIRMENT OF THE ADRENERGIC INNERVATION OF NTS

After discovering that destructive lesions of NTS in cat can produce chronic labile hypertension, attempts were made to determine if imbalances of neurotransmitters within the same nucleus can also produce abnormal regulation of the arterial pressure. The NTS and adjacent regions of the dorsal medulla are richly innervated by catecholamine containing neurons (Chiba and Doba, 1975, 1976; Dahlström and Fuxe, 1964; Fuxe *et al.*, 1970; Palkovits and Jacobowitz, 1974; Swanson and Hartman, 1975; Torack *et al.*, 1973; Ungerstedt, 1971). The principal noradrenergic innervation appears to arise from neurons of the so-called A2 group of Dahlström and Fuxe (1964) whose cell bodies lie in medial and commissural portions of the NTS (Dahlström and Fuxe, 1964; Swanson and Hartman, 1975; Torack *et al.*, 1973). The A2 neurons have been presumed, largely on pharmacological evidence, to exert a vasodepressor function, possibly by facilitating baroreceptor reflexes (De Jong and Nijkamp, 1975, 1976; De Jong *et al.*, 1975; Finch *et al.*, 1975; Haeusler, 1974; Helse and Kroneberg, 1973; Henning and Robinson, 1971; Kobinger and Wallard, 1972a,b; Korner *et al.*, 1974; Nijkamp and De Jong, 1975; Srivastava *et al.*, 1973).

By immunocytochemical techniques using specific antibodies to the enzyme tyrosine hydroxylase (TH) (Pickel *et al.*, 1976, 1977, 1979), the enzyme catalyzing the rate-limiting step in catecholamine biosynthesis, we have been able to assess the distribution of A2 neurons in the rat brain. We have also been able to examine the neurons by electron microscopy and demonstrate that these neurons are richly innervated by fibers containing tryptophan hydroxylase (and are hence serotonergic), as well as by processes from neurons containing the peptides enkephalin and substance P (Pickel *et al.*, 1977, 1979).

A. Effect of Electrolytic Lesions of A2

In the chronically instrumented, freely moving rat, an electrolytic lesion that destroyed the bulk of the A2 neurons resulted in a characteristic cardiovascular syndrome (Reis *et al.*, 1979). After a transient elevation of arterial pressure, lasting about 24 hours, rats developed chronic lability of their arterial pressure without hypertension and without any substantial change in average values or lability of the heart rate (Fig. 7 and Table I). The lability of arterial pressure appears permanent and is associated with some exaggeration of the reactivity of the pressure during spontaneous behaviors, or in response to emotional stimuli. A2 lesions abolish the baroreceptor reflex and, as evidence that those cells largely innervate NTS, result in a reduction of the activity of the marker

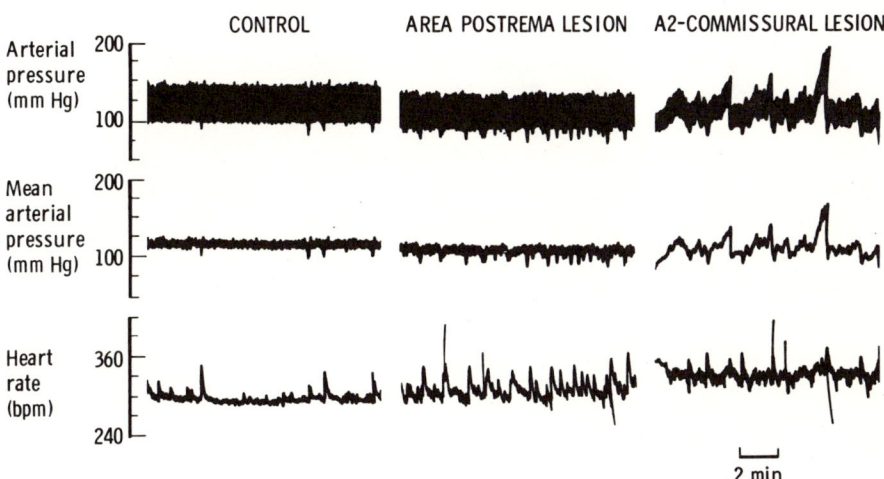

Fig. 7. Lability of arterial pressure produced by electrolytic lesions of A2-commissural area in the rat 4 days prior to recording pressure, as compared with rats with lesion of area postrema and an unoperated control. (From Talman *et al.*, 1980.)

TABLE 1.

Comparison of Effects of Electrolytic Lesions of A2 Area or Microinjection of 6-OHDA into NTS on Cardiovascular Function and in DBH Activity in NTS

	A2 Lesions		6-OHDA [b]	
Property [a]	Controls	A2 Lesions	Controls	Lesions
MAP (mmHg)	118 ± 2.5	118 ± 5.9 (ns)	108 ± 2.0	107 ± 4.0 (ns)
$S.D._{MAP}$ (mmHg)	6.0 ± 0.5	13.0 ± 1.3 **	5.8 ± 0.4	15.1 ± 1.8 ***
$\dfrac{S.D._{MAP}}{MAP} \times 100$	5.1	11.0	5.4	14.1
HR (bpm)	366 ± 10	354 ± 16 (ns)	342 ± 14	330 ± 12 (ns)
$S.D._{HR}$	28.4 ± 3.5	20.5 ± 5.4 (ns)	25.4 ± 4.2	18.1 ± 1.4 *
$\dfrac{S.D._{HR}}{HR} \times 100$	7.8	5.7	7.4	5.5
Baroreceptor reflex	Present	Absent	Present	Present
DBH activity (% of control)	100	57 ± 7 **	100	40 ± 3 **

[a] MAP, mean arterial pressure; HR, heart rate; bpm, beats per minute; S.D., standard deviation; DBH, dopamine-β-hydroxylase. All values expressed as mean $\pm$ SEM. ns, not significant; *, $p < .05$; **, $p < .01$; ***, $p < .001$.

[b] Data from Nathan *et al.* (1978).

enzyme dopamine-β-hydroxylase (DBH) in the NTS, to about 50% of control. Morphometric analysis has established a direct correlation between the number of A2 neurons destroyed and the amount of lability produced (Reis *et al.*, 1979).

Destruction of the terminals of noradrenergic innervation to NTS by administration of the drug 6-OHDA bilaterally into NTS produces an almost identical syndrome (Reis *et al.*, 1979; Snyder *et al.*, 1978b). Within 24 hours after administration of an optimal dose (4 μg in 1 μl), rats develop chronic lability of the arterial pressure without hypertension or changes in heart rate (Fig. 8 and Table I). DBH activity is reduced to 40% of control. Unlike A2 lesions, however, destruction of the terminals in NTS does not abolish baroreceptor reflexes.

B. The Function of A2 Neurons in the Control of Arterial Pressure

It is evident from these studies that A2 neurons function in regulating the circulation. The major deficit produced by lesions in the cell bodies or terminals is the production of a profound lability of the arterial pressure without hypertension and exaggerated reactivity of the arterial

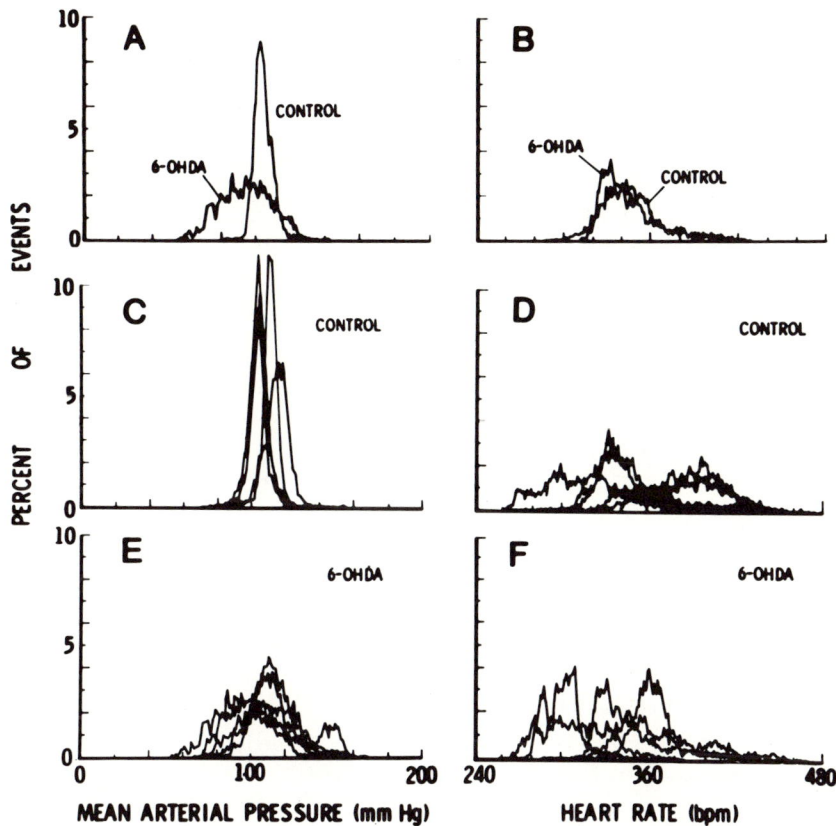

Fig. 8. Frequency distribution curves of mean arterial pressure and heart rate in control and 6-OHDA treated rats. Panels A and B represent changes in the same animal before and 3 days after treatment. Panels C and D are an overlay of five control rats from 4 days after vehicle (0.8 mg/ml ascorbic acid) was microinjected into NTS. Panels E and F are an overlay of five rats 4 days after 6-OHDA (4 μg in 1 μl) was injected into NTS bilaterally. Note increased lability of arterial pressure into 6-OHDA treatment.

pressure. The similarity between the syndromes produced either by lesions of the cell bodies or by terminals of A2 cells is striking (Table I). The only difference between the two types of lesions is that the destruction of the cell bodies results in the disappearance of baroreceptor reflexes, probably a consequence of lesions of neurons other than A2 or of afferents projecting medially (Chiba and Doba, 1975, 1976; Miura and Reis, 1969, 1972). Preservation of baroreceptor reflexes in the face of lability, following lesions of the terminals by 6-OHDA, demonstrates that (1) lability is not due to loss of baroreceptor afferents, (2) the primary baroreceptor afferents are not catecholaminergic, and (3) the lability produced by lesions of the A2 cells themselves is unlikely to be due to secondary changes in projections of A2 neurons to regions other than NTS.

Our findings suggest that the catecholaminergic innervation of A2, probably mediated by norepinephrine, serves to stabilize the arterial pressure by acting in concert with baroreceptors. The fact that deficiencies in this system lead to lability of arterial pressure is of interest since lability of blood pressure is frequently an early sign of hypertension in man. The results, therefore, indicate that an abnormality in a biochemically selective system of the brain can produce conditions that may favor the development of hypertension at a later date.

IV. SUMMARY AND CONCLUSIONS

There is new interest in a possible role of the sympathetic nervous system, the brain, and central monoamine neurons in the expression and even the initiation of hypertension. The application of research strategies and techniques of the neurosciences to what, heretofore, had been primarily a cardiovascular research area, has been fruitful. Systematic investigations have led to the development of a model of neurogenic hypertension of central origin, that produced by bilateral electrolytic lesions of the nucleus tractus solitarii (NTS), and the demonstration that biochemical abnormalities of the catecholamine innervation of the region can produce lability of blood pressure. Of particular interest has been the observation that lesions of NTS in the cat lead to exaggerated responses to environmental and emotional stimuli. This finding raises the possibility that, for emotional stress to lead to hypertension, a concomitant abnormality of baroreflex integration must be present. Investigations of the neurobiology of monoamine neurons of the brain, which regulate arterial pressure, may be an important frontier in linking molecular defects to the development of hyperactivity in the sympathetic nervous system. These studies have established the fact that imbalances within cardiovascular centers of the brain can lead to hypertension and that neurochemical dysfunction can predispose to conditions of the circulation which may contribute to the development of fixed hypertension.

ACKNOWLEDGMENTS

The author wishes to thank Drs. R. Dampney, N. Doba, T. H. Joh, M. Kumada, M. Nathan, D. Snyder, and W. Talman whose collaborative efforts form the basis of this report. This research was supported by grants from the National Institutes of Health and the National Aeronautics and Space Administration.

REFERENCES

Alexander, R. S. (1946). Tonic and reflex functions of medullary sympathetic cardio-vascular centers. *J. Neurophysiol.* **9**, 205–217.

Amer, M. S., Gomoll, A. W., Perhach, J. L., Jr., Ferguson, H. C., and McKinney, G. R. (1974). Aberrations of cyclic nucleotide metabolism in the hearts and vessels of hypertensive rats. *Proc. Natl. Acad. Sci. U.S.A.* **71**, 4930–4934.

Amer, M. S., Doba, N., and Reis, D. J. (1975). Changes in cyclic nucleotide metabolism in aorta and heart of neurogenically hypertensive rats: possible trigger mecha-nism of hypertension. *Proc. Natl. Acad. Sci. U.S.A.* **72**, 2135–2139.

Brody, M. J., Fink, G. D., Buggy, J., Haywood, J. R., Gordon, F., Knvepfer, M. M., Mahoney, L., and Johnson, K. (1979). Critical role of the anteroventral third ven-tricle (AV3V) region in development and maintenance of experimental hyperten-sion. *In* "Nervous System and Hypertension" (P. Meyer and H. Schmitt, eds.), pp. 76–84. Wiley Flammarion, Paris and New York.

Chalmers, J. P. (1975). Brain amines and models of experimental hypertension. *Circ. Res.* **36**, 469–480.

Chiba, T., and Doba, N. (1975). The synaptic structure of catecholaminergic axon varicosities in the dorso-medial portion of the nucleus tractus solitarius of the cat: possible roles in the regulation of cardiovascular reflexes. *Brain Res.* **84**, 31–46.

Chiba, T., and Doba, N. (1976). Catecholaminergic axo-axonic synapses in the nucleus of the tractus solitarius (pars commissuralis) of the cat: possible relation to presynaptic regulation of baroreceptor reflexes. *Brain Res.* **102**, 255–265.

Cottle, M. K. (1964). Degeneration studies of primary afferents of IXth and Xth cranial nerves in the cat. *J. Comp. Neurol.* **122**, 329–345.

Cowley, A. W., Jr., Liard, J. F., and Guyton, A. C. (1973). Role of the baroreceptor reflex in daily control of arterial blood pressure and other variables in dogs. *Circ. Res.* **32**, 564–576.

Dahlström, A., and Fuxe, K. (1964). Evidence for the existence of monoamine-containing neurons in the central nervous system. I. Demonstration of monoamines in the cell bodies of brain stem neurons. *Acta Physiol. Scand., Suppl.* **232**, 1–55.

Dampney, R. A., Kumada, M., and Reis, D. J. (1979). Central neural mechanisms of the cerebral ischemic response: characterization, effect of brainstem and cranial nerve transections, and simulation by electrical stimulation of restricted regions of medulla oblongata in rabbit. *Circ. Res.* **44**, 48–62.

De Jong, W., and Nijkamp, F. P. (1975). Hypotensive action of noradrenaline and α-methylnoradrenaline in the area of the nucleus tractus solitarii in the rat brainstem. *In* "Central Action of Drugs in Blood Pressure Regulation" (D. S. Davies, and J. L. Reid, eds.), pp. 179–180. Univ. Park Press, Baltimore, Maryland.

De Jong, W., and Nijkamp, F. P. (1976). Centrally induced hypotension and brady-cardia after administration of α-methylnoradrenaline into the area of the nucleus tractus solitarii of the rat. *Br. J. Pharmacol.* **58**, 593–598.

De Jong, W., Zandberg, P., and Bohus, B. (1975). Central inhibitory noradrenergic cardiovascular control. *In* "Hormones, Homeostasis and the Brain" (W. H. Gispen, T. B. van Wilmersma Greidanus, B. Bohus, and D. DeWied, eds.), Progress in Brain Research, Vol. 42, pp. 285–298. Am. Elsevier, New York.

De Jong, W., Provoost, A. P., and Shapiro, A. P., eds. (1977). "Hypertension and Brain Mechanisms," Progress in Brain Research, Vol. 47. Elsevier, Amsterdam.

De Quattro, V., and Miura, Y. (1973). Neurogenic factors in human hypertension: Mechanism or myth? *Am. J. Med.* **55**, 362–378.

Dickenson, C. J. (1965). "Neurogenic Hypertension." Blackwell, Oxford.

Doba, N., and Reis, D. J. (1973). Acute fulminating neurogenic hypertension produced by brainstem lesions in the rat. *Circ. Res.* **32**, 584–593.

Doba, N., and Reis, D. J. (1974). Role of central and peripheral adrenergic mechanisms in neurogenic hypertension produced by brainstem lesions in rats. *Circ. Res.* **34**, 293–301.

Farris, E. J., Yeakel, E. H., and Medoff, H. S. (1945). Development of hypertension in emotional gray Norway rats after air blasting. *Am. J. Physiol.* **144**, 331–336.

Finch, L., Buckingham, R. E., Moore, R. A., and Bucher, T. J. (1975). Evidence for a central α-sympathetic action of clonidine in the rat. *J. Pharm. Pharmacol.* **27**, 181–186.

Folkow, B. (1971). The haemodynamic consequences of adaptive structural changes of the resistance vessels in hypertension. *Clin. Sci.* **41**, 1–12.

Folkow, B., and Rubenstein, E. H. (1966). Cardiovascular effects of acute and chronic stimulation of the hypothalamic defense area in the rat. *Acta Physiol. Scand.* **68**, 48–57.

Fuxe, K., Hokfelt, T., Jonsson, G., and Ungerstedt, U. (1970). Fluorescence microscopy in neuroanatomy. *In* "Contemporary Research Methods in Neuroanatomy" (W. J. H. Nauta and S. O. E. Ebbesson, eds.), pp. 275–314. Springer-Verlag, Berlin and New York.

Genest, J., Koiw, E., and Kuchel, O., eds. (1977). "Hypertension." McGraw-Hill, New York.

Haeusler, G. (1974). Clonidine-induced inhibition of sympathetic nerve activity: no indication for a central presynaptic or an indirect sympathomimetic mode of action. *Naunyn-Schmiedeberg's Arch. Pharmacol.* **286**, 97–111.

Harris, A. H., and Brady, J. W. (1974). Animal learning; visceral and autonomic conditioning. *Annu. Rev. Psychol.* **25**, 107–143.

Helse, A., and Kroneberg, G. (1973). Central nervous α-adrenergic receptors and the mode of action of α-methyldopa. *Naunyn-Schmiedeberg's Arch. Pharmacol.* **279**, 285–300.

Henning, M., and Robinson, A. (1971). Evidence that the hypotensive action of methyldopa is mediated by central actions of methylnoradrenaline. *J. Pharm. Pharmacol.* **23**, 407–411.

Henry, J. P., Stephens, P. M., and Axelrod, J. (1971). Effect of psychosocial stimulation on the enzymes involved in the biosynthesis and metabolism of noradrenaline and adrenaline. *Psychosom. Med.* **33**, 227–237.

Herd, J. A., Morse, W. H., Kelleher, R. T., and Jones, L. G. (1969). Arterial hypertension in the squirrel monkey during behavioral experiments. *Am. J. Physiol.* **217**, 24–29.

Hilton, S. M. (1963). Inhibition of baroreceptor reflexes on hypothalamic stimulation. *J. Physiol. (London)* **165**, 56–57.

Julius, S., and Esler, M. D., eds. (1976). "The Nervous System in Arterial Hypertension." Thomas, Springfield, Illinois.

Kobinger, W., and Walland, A. W. (1972a). Evidence for a central activation of a vagal cardiodepressor reflex by clonidine. *Eur. J. Pharmacol.* **19**, 203–209.

Kobinger, W., and Walland, A. W. (1972b). Facilitation of vagal reflex bradycardia by an action of clonidine on central α-receptors. *Eur. J. Pharmacol.* **19**, 210–217.

Koch-Weser, J. (1973). Sympathetic activity in essential hypertension. *N. Engl. J. Med.* **288**, 627–628.

Korner, P. I., Oliver, J. R., Sleight, P., Chalmers, J. P., and Robinson, J. S. (1974). Effects of clonidine on the baroreceptor-heart rate reflex and on single aortic baroreceptor fibre discharge. *Eur. J. Pharmacol.* **28**, 189–198.

Kumada, M., Dampney, A. L., and Reis, D. J. (1979). Profound hypotension and abolition of the vasomotor component of the cerebral ischemic response produced by restricted lesions of medulla oblongata: Relationship to the so-called tonic vasomotor center. *Circ. Res.* **44**, 63–70.

Lamprecht, F., Williams, R. B., and Kopin, I. J. (1973). Serum dopamine-beta-hydroxylase during development of immobilization-induced hypertension. *Endocrinology* **92**, 953–956.

Laragh, J. H., ed. (1974). "Hypertension Manual." Yorke Med. Books, New York.

Littler, W. A., Honour, A. J., Sleight P., and Stott E. D. (1972). Continuous recording of direct arterial pressure and electrocardiogram in unrestricted man. *Br. Med. J.* **3**, 76–78.

Littler, W. A., Honour, A. J., Pugsley, D. J., and Sleight, P. (1976). The use of 24 hour blood pressure monitoring in the diagnosis and management of difficult hypertensive problems. *Postgrad. Med. J., Suppl.* **7**, 119–122.

Louis, W. J., Doyle, A. E., and Anavekar, S. (1973). Plasma norepinephrine levels in essential hypertension. *N. Engl. J. Med.* **288**, 599–601.

Mendlowitz, M., and Vlachakis, N. D. (1976). The catecholamines in essential hypertension. *Am. Heart J.* **91**, 378–382.

Miura, M., and Reis, D. J. (1969). Termination and secondary projections of carotid sinus nerve in the cat brain stem. *Am. J. Physiol.* **217**, 142–153.

Miura, M., and Reis, D. J. (1972). The role of the solitary and paramedian reticular nuclei in mediating cardiovascular reflex responses from carotid baro- and chemoreceptors. *J. Physiol. (London)* **223**, 525–548.

Nathan, M. A., and Reis, D. J. (1977). Chronic labile hypertension produced by lesions of the nucleus tractus solitarii in the cat. *Circ. Res.* **40**, 72–81.

Nathan, M. A., Tucker, L. W., Severini, W. H., and Reis, D. J. (1978). Enhancement of conditioned arterial pressure responses in cats after brainstem lesions. *Science* **201**, 71–73.

Nijkamp, F. P., and De Jong, W. (1975). α-Methylnoradrenaline induced hypotension and bradycardia after administration into the area of the nucleus tractus solitarii. *Eur. J. Pharmacol.* **32**, 361–364.

Onesti, G., Fernandes, M., and Kim, K. E., eds. (1976). "Regulation of Blood Pressure by the Central Nervous System." Grune & Stratton, New York.

Palkovits, M., and Jacobowitz, D. M. (1974). Topographic atlas of catecholamine and acetylcholinesterase-containing neurons in the rat brain. II. Hindbrain (mesencephalon, rhombencephalon). *J. Comp. Neurol.* **157**, 29–42.

Pickel, V. M., Joh, T. H., and Reis, D. J. (1976). Monoamine-synthesizing enzymes in central dopaminergic, noradrenergic and serotonergic neurons. Immunocytochemical localization by light and electron microscopy. *J. Histochem. Cytochem.* **24**, 792–806.

Pickel, V. M., Joh, T. H., and Reis, D. J. (1977). A serotonergic innervation of noradrenergic neurons in nucleus locus coeruleus: demonstration by immunocytochemical localization of the transmitter specific enzymes tyrosine and tryptophan hydroxylase. *Brain Res.* **131**, 197–214.

Pickel, V. M., Joh, T. H., Reis, D. J., Leeman, S. E., and Miller, R. J. (1979). Electron microscopic localization of substance P and enkephalin in axon terminals related to dendrites of catecholaminergic neurons. *Brain Res.* **160**, 387–400.

Pickering, G. (1968). "High Blood Pressure." Grune & Stratton, New York.

Reis, D. J., and Cuenod, M. (1964). Tonic influence of rostral brain structures on pressure regulatory mechanisms in the cat. *Science* 145, 64–65.

Reis, D. J., and Doba, N. (1974). The central nervous system and neurogenic hypertension. *Prog. Cardiovasc. Dis.* 17, 51–71.

Reis, D. J., Joh, T. H., Nathan, M. A., Renaud, B., Snyder, D. W., and Talman, W. T. (1979). The nucleus tractus solitarii, its catecholaminergic innervation, and the normal and abnormal control of arterial pressure. *In* "Perspectives in Nephrology and Hyptertension" (H. Schmitt and P. Meyer, eds.), pp. 147–164. Wiley, New York.

Sivertsson, R. (1970). The hemodynamic importance of structural vascular changes in essential hypertension. *Acta Physiol. Scand., Suppl.* 343, 1–56.

Snyder, D. W., Doba, N., and Reis, D. J. (1978a). Regional distribution of blood flow during arterial hypertension produced by lesion of the nucleus tractus solitarii in rats. *Circ. Res.* 42, 87–91.

Snyder, D. W., Nathan, M. A., and Reis, D. J. (1978b). Chronic lability of arterial pressure produced by selective denervation of the catecholamine innervation of the nucleus tractus solitarii in rat. *Circ. Res.* 43, 662–671.

Srivastava, R. K., Kalshrestah, V. K., Singh, N., and Bhargava, K. P. (1973). Central cardiovascular effects of intracerebroventricular propranolol. *Eur. J. Pharmacol.* 21, 222–229.

Swanson, L. W., and Hartman, B. K. (1975). The central adrenergic system. An immunofluorescence study of the location of cell bodies and their efferent connections in the rat utilizing dopamine-β-hydroxylase as a marker. *J. Comp. Neurol.* 163, 467–506.

Talman, W. T., Snyder, D. W., and Reis, D. J. (1980). Chronic lability of arterial pressure produced by destruction of A2 catecholamine neurons in rat brainstem. *Circ. Res.* (in press).

Torack, R. M., Stranahan, P., and Hartman, B. K. (1973). The role of norepinephrine in the function of the area postrema. I. Immunofluorescent localization of dopamine-beta-hydroxylase and electron microscopy. *Brain Res.* 61, 235–252.

Ungerstedt, U. (1971). I. Stereotaxic mapping of the monoamine pathway in the rat brain. *Acta Physiol. Scand., Suppl.* 367, 1–48.

Zanchetti, A., ed. (1972). "Neural and Psychological Mechanisms in Cardiovascular Disease." Il Ponte, Milan.

5

The Molecular Mechanisms for the Long-Term Transsynaptic Regulation of Adrenal Medullary Function

E. Costa

ISBN 0-12-360850-3

I. INTRODUCTION

A number of biochemical processes that regulate the cardiocirculatory function are modulated by the interaction of putative neurotransmitters with specific receptors. Catecholamines are prominent among the neurotransmitters involved in this regulation. They interact with specific receptors in the target cell membranes, following their extracellular release from stores located in axon terminals or in chromaffin cells of adrenal medulla. Since, by the latter mechanism, catecholamines are secreted into the bloodstream, they can simultaneously affect the receptors located on the membrane of a great number of target cells. Because of the great functional significance of this secretion on cardiocirculatory regulation, not only is the synthesis rate of medullary catecholamines increased during a persistent increase of secretion, but also new synthesis of tyrosine hydroxylase (TH) molecules takes place (Chuang and Costa, 1974; Chuang *et al.*, 1975). The regulation of TH behaves as if it were a specific mechanism which oversees the constant fullness of the stores of catecholamines in adrenal medulla. The efficiency of this long-term regulation of TH biosynthesis is such that transsynaptic regulation of protein synthesis in adrenal medulla has become a model, not only in studying regulation of catecholamine stores, but also in investigating how nuclear function can be regulated via an activation of cell membrane receptors. The selection of the adrenal medulla as a model for the latter studies was prompted by the realization that adrenal medulla is formed by a homogeneous cell population, that it has only one type of afferent neuron, and that changes in its messenger RNA biosynthesis can be evoked by stimulating nicotinic receptors (Guidotti and Costa, 1977).

The secretion of catecholamines from adrenal medulla is regulated transsynaptically by the release of acetylcholine (Guidotti and Costa, 1974). This neurotransmitter acts on muscarinic and nicotinic receptors located on the membrane of chromaffin cells. The activation of nicotinic receptors initiates and regulates exocytosis and exerts trophic influences. Two actions on medullary cells will be considered: a short-term Ca^{2+}-dependent secretion of catecholamines, and a long-term Ca^{2+}-independent trophic action (Guidotti and Costa, 1974 ; Guidotti *et al.*, 1975a). Both of these actions depend on the activation of nicotinic receptors. At this time, it would be difficult to ascribe a particular medullary function to the medullary muscarinic receptors. However, secretion of catecholamines may not be the only function of chromaffin cells. Preliminary evidence is emerging that indicates that splanchnic nerves and medullary cells also store an enkephalinlike peptide, which may function as a secondary putative neurotransmitter (DiGiulio *et al.*, 1978). Perhaps muscarinic receptors modulate the release and synthesis of this enkeph-alinlike polypeptide.

The amount of acetylcholine that is released into chromaffin cell membranes from the terminal axon of the splanchnic neurons that innervate chromaffin cells is determined by the coordinated activity of a number of brain neurons, which are connected to each other in a very precise way. Within this neuronal network there is a precise logic whereby, when a high release rate of acetylcholine persists for a long time, precise instructions are given to the nucleus of the postsynaptic chromaffin cells to change the rate of RNA metabolism, in order to produce enough TH to sustain high rates of catecholamine release. That the site where this logic resides is the nicotinic synapse is inferred from experiments showing that injections of the nicotinic receptor agonist to rats with denervated adrenal medulla elicited a long-term trophic action on adrenal medulla (Hanbauer and Guidotti, 1975), as expressed by an accumulation of newly synthesized TH molecules (Chuang and Costa, 1974; Chuang *et al.*, 1975).

This chapter will discuss the mechanism whereby the activation of nicotinic receptors can bring about the appropriate and specific increase in the synthesis of messenger RNA, to make possible a transsynaptic induction of TH. The trophic response will be discussed in terms of the increase in TH activity (Thoenen *et al.*, 1969a,b) and in the biosynthesis rate of this enzyme (Chuang *et al.*, 1975).

II. MECHANISMS FOR LONG-TERM TRANSSYNAPTIC REGULATION

A. Muscarinic and Nicotinic Receptors and the Function of Adrenal Medulla

Axelrod and colleagues (Thoenen *et al.*, 1969a,b; Axelrod, 1971) reported that the activity of TH can be regulated transsynaptically, via changes in RNA transcription and protein synthesis (Chuang and Costa, 1976). From these studies, the cholinergic synapses of the medulla emerged as a convergence point for the regulation of protein synthesis and catecholamine secretion in chromaffin cells. By itself, this convergence raised the question of how to dissociate the regulation of two phenomena that depend on the function of one type of synapse. This problem was elucidated by *in vivo* (Chuang and Costa, 1974; Chuang *et al.*, 1975; Guidotti and Costa, 1974a, 1977; Guidotti *et al.*, 1975a) and *in vitro* experiments using rat adrenal medulla and primary cultures of bovine chromaffin cells (Kumakura *et al.*, 1978), respectively.

Physiological experiments and work done with cultured chromaffin cells from bovine adrenal medulla indicate that stimulation of muscarinic receptors located on chromaffin cell membranes fails to elicit catecholamine secretion. Moreover, the stimulation of muscarinic receptors fails to increase the 3′,5′-cyclic adenosine monophosphate (cAMP) content of adrenal medulla; whereas, the cAMP content of chromaffin cells is conspicuously elevated by the stimulation of nicotinic receptors both *in vitro* and *in vivo* (Guidotti *et al.,* 1975a). In contrast, the stimulation of muscarinic receptors is associated with an increase in the medullary concentration of 3′,5′-guanosine monophosphate (cGMP), at least *in vivo* (Guidotti *et al.,* 1975a). This response is facilitated by hexamethonium but is blocked by atropine (Guidotti *et al.,* 1975a). These experiments suggest that the stimulation of nicotinic receptors regulates two responses: a secretory response which is cAMP-independent, and another response which becomes evident only following a persistent stimulation and depends on the activation of adenylate cyclase (Guidotti and Costa, 1974b; Guidotti *et al.,* 1975b). The stimulation of muscarinic receptors increases guanylate cyclase activity and causes an accumulation of cGMP, following persistent stimulation (Guidotti *et al.,* 1975a). It is not yet understood if cholinergic receptor agonists activate cyclase because there is a direct membrane coupling between cyclases and cholinergic receptors, or because there is a direct membrane coupling between cyclases and cholinergic receptors since more complex mechanisms are operative (Guidotti and Costa, 1974a).

Experimentally, an activation of adenylate cyclase by acetylcholine (ACh) or other nicotinic receptor agonists could be shown with slices of adrenal medulla (Guidotti and Costa, 1974a); however, when cell-free systems were used, the cholinomimetics failed to stimulate adenylate cyclase (Guidotti and Costa, 1974a). This finding prompted the question of whether or not this increase in medullary cAMP content was an effect related to the stimulation of nicotinic receptors (Thoenen and Otten, 1975). The exact membrane location of adenylate cyclase on the coupling between receptor and enzyme is not understood at this time. Hence, is was possible to speculate (Thoenen and Otten, 1975) that the catecholamines, released from their storage site, could activate adrenergic receptors located in the chromaffin cell membrane and thereby increase the activity of cellular adenylate cyclase (Otten *et al.,* 1974a). Direct experiments were carried out with catecholamine receptor blockers. These drugs failed to block the increase of cAMP content elicited by a direct or indirect activation of nicotinic receptors (Guidotti *et al.,* 1975b). That the release of catecholamines is unrelated to the cAMP content of adrenal medulla, is suggested by the lack of catecholamine release elicited by 8-Br-cAMP added to primary cell culture of chromaffin cells ($10M$) in the presence of 1.5 mM Ca^{2+}.

B. Trophic Changes Elicited in Chromaffin Cells by Nicotinic Receptor Agonists

In the medulla, the onset of cAMP increase depends on nicotinic receptor stimulation, but the duration of this increase is unrelated to the duration of nicotinic receptor stimulation. During persistent stimulation lasting 1 hr or more, the medullary cAMP content returns to normal within 60 to 90 min, although the secretory response is still operative (Hanbauer et al., 1975). This uncoupling between the duration of two responses, which depend on the activation of the same receptor, was explained by the activation of cAMP catabolism which selectively nullifies the cAMP accumulation (Guidotti and Costa, 1977). Previous reports by other laboratories had indicated that the stimulation of medullary nicotinic receptors triggered a long-term change in nuclear metabolic activity, leading to an induction of several protein constituents of the chromaffin cells including TH (Thoenen et al., 1969b; Axelrod, 1971; Thoenen and Otten, 1974, 1975; Otten et al., 1974a,b).

The molecular nature of the events by which the binding of a neurotransmitter to its receptor (located in the cell membrane of postsynaptic cells) modifies the metabolism in the nucleus is still poorly understood. There appear to be two classes of mechanisms that are activated in the postsynaptic cell, as a result of the interactions of a transmitter with its receptor. One class concerns the regulation of ion fluxes. Hence, the recognition site of the transmitter located in the outer part of the membrane is thought to be coupled directly with an ionophore mechanism. Although the precise relationship existing between the transmitter receptor and ionophore is not known, it can be assumed that the binding of the transmitter to the recognition site triggers a conformational change in a specific ionophore, leading to a change in the membrane permeability to a specific ion. The dependence of the catecholamine release from stimulation of nicotinic receptors and the strict requirement of Ca^{2+} for catecholamine release lends credence to the hypothesis that a Ca^{2+} ionophore might be operative in the process whereby nicotinic receptor activation releases catecholamines from medullary stores. When dealing with Ca^{2+} ionophore, allowance has to be made for the participation of a specific protein (calmodulin) which probably mediates the Ca^{2+} response in several types of cells (Cheung et al., 1975; Bromstrom et al., 1975; Klee, 1977). Different types of Ca^{2+} binding protein have been identified; that in red blood cells (Gopinath and Vincenzi, 1977) appears to differ immunologically from the calmodulin of brain (I. Hanbauer, personal communication).

The second class of mechanisms concerns the activation of second messenger responses. In the medulla, a stimulation of the nicotinic receptors triggers a process that leads to the production of cAMP as a second messenger molecule inside of the chromaffin cell. In mammalian cells, a specific class of protein kinases is the universal receptor for cAMP (Krebs, 1972). These kinases are present in many cell compartments, including the membranes; when cAMP increases, it catalyzes phosphorylation of proteins in various cell compartments, including a phosphorylation of membrane protein. However, when the cytosol concentration of this second messenger in chromaffin cells reaches a critical value and the duration of this increase exceeds a certain limit, a sequence of biochemical reactions occurs, which ultimately modifies nuclear metabolism (Kurosawa et al., 1976a). How these changes occurring in cytosol trigger a change in the metabolic properties of the nucleus is still not understood. However, the translocation of protein kinase catalytic subunits from cytosol to the nucleus is now being considered (Guidotti and Costa, 1977; Kurosawa et al., 1976a; Chuang et al., 1976, 1977).

While the function of receptors coupled with ionophores appears to be a typical modality to trigger the immediate and transitory synaptic responses elicited by neurotransmitters, the second messenger response may be operative in more stable responses such as the trophic response. Second messengers were first described as a mechanism that mediates the metabolic responses of hormones in nonneuronal tissues (Sutherland and Rall, 1960). Only after the pioneer work of Sutherland and colleagues, on beta receptors, and the early studies (Robison et al., 1971) on the regulation of adenylate cyclase of the pineal gland by catecholamines (Weiss and Costa, 1967), has cAMP been considered to be operative as an intracellular mediator for the action of neurotransmitters. Chromaffin cells are regulated by only one type of neuron. It is conceivable that the ionophore, which is activated by the interaction between the transmitter and the postsynaptic receptor of chromaffin cells, triggers exocytosis and catecholamine secretions. However, with persistent receptor stimulation, in some unknown way, the adenylate cyclase also becomes coupled to the responses elicited by the activation of nicotinic receptors. Through this functional interaction, the nicotinic receptor may regulate chromaffin cell trophism and trigger the long-term metabolic responses, including the increase in synthesis of mRNA specific for TH. That cyclic nucleotides in chromaffin cells may function in the regulation of cell trophism, is supported by the evidence that

8-Br-cAMP added to the primary cultures of chromaffin cells (Kumakura *et al.*, 1978) or to neuroblastoma cell cultures (R. Hollenbeck, unpublished observations) causes a long-term induction of TH. As mentioned earlier, the addition of 8-Br-cAMP fails to release catecholamines because it fails to activate the Ca^{2+} ionophore coupled with exocytosis. That an activation of Ca^{2+} ionophore is coupled with the activation of acetylcholine receptors had been proposed also in other neuronal systems.

C. Transsynaptic Induction of TH: A Model to Study Molecular Mechanisms Whereby Synapses Regulate Cell Trophism

Axelrod and colleagues (Thoenen *et al.*, 1969b; Axelrod, 1971) reported that medullary TH activity increases after the injection of nicotinic receptor agonists, or when the activity of cholinergic neurons innervating the medulla increases. This finding has been confirmed (Costa and Guidotti, 1973; Costa *et al.*, 1974, 1975a,c). In addition, a cascade of events was shown to occur, following a persistent cholinergic stimulation (Guidotti *et al.*, 1973); this cascade began with an increase in cAMP, followed by an activation of protein kinase and an increase in RNA transcription and protein synthesis (Chuang and Costa, 1974, 1976; Chuang *et al.*, 1975; Thoenen *et al.*, 1969b; Guidotti and Costa, 1973). The transcription process was terminated within 8–10 hr following the stimulus application (Chuang and Costa, 1974; Guidotti *et al.*, 1975b; Guidotti and Costa, 1973), while the increase in protein synthesis lasted for various time periods which depended on the $T_{1/2}$ of the mRNA. The increase of TH synthesis lasted about 30 hr, probably the life span of the mRNA. With the exception of the injection of nicotinic receptor agonists, however, all other stimuli failed to increase the TH activity when applied after adrenal denervation (Guidotti and Costa, 1974a; Hanbauer and Guidotti, 1975; Axelrod, 1971; Costa *et al.*, 1975c; Thoenen *et al.*, 1973). Since all the inducing stimuli act via the cholinergic synapses, the induction of medullary TH was termed "transsynaptic." However, the evidence produced by Axelrod and associates and by Thoenen *et al.* (1973) left open the possibility that, when medullary TH activity is increased, the number of TH molecules may not increase; but the increase in TH activity is due to the lack of formation of an endogenous inhibitor. This possibility was negated by immunotitration studies showing that the increase in medullary TH was due to an increase in the number of TH molecules (Joh *et al.*, 1973). Moreover, in our laboratory, using specific antibodies and pulse injections of radioactive amino acids, it was shown that the amount of radioactivity incorporated into TH increases from 6 to 36 hr after a stimulus that induces TH (Chuang and Costa, 1974, 1976; Chuang et al., 1975; Guidotti et al., 1975b; Costa et al., 1975d). The rates of synthesis and degradation of TH were estimated by measuring the radioactivity incorporated into TH purified immunochromatographically after a 90 min pulse with [³H]leucine (Chuang and Costa, 1974; Chuang et al., 1975). The increment in TH activity occurs a few hours after the incorporation of radioactive leucine into immunoreactive TH has occurred. TH activity becomes detectable at 12 hr, reaches a maximum at 24 hr, and virtually remains at this maximum for about 4 days (Fig. 1). After 4 days, it begins to decline, and on the day 11 following the stimulus, the increased activity is no longer detectable. Thus, after induction the $T_{1/2}$ of TH increase is about 3 days (Fig. 1).

To measure whether or not the rate of degradation of medullary TH changes during the transsynaptic induction, the rats received pulse of [³H]leucine 48 hr after the stimulus, and the decay of the radioactivity incorporated into TH was measured during a time in which the TH content virtually remained at a steady state level (Guidotti et al., 1975b). It was found that the decay of the specific radioactivity followed first order kinetics and had a $T_{1/2}$ of 68 hr (Guidotti et al., 1975b). When a group of untreated rats, run in parallel, was tested, the characteristics of the TH specific radioactivity was comparable. A strong indication that during TH induction the TH degradation failed to change, was obtained by double-labeling experiments, which indicated that TH has a turnover time of about 100 hr (Chuang and Costa, 1974). This turnover time agrees with the decay of TH activity shown in Fig. 1 and with the $T_{1/2}$ of 68 hr, obtained by measuring the decay rate of TH specific radioactivity (Chuang and Costa, 1976; Guidotti et al., 1975b).

D. Participation of cAMP in Transsynaptic Regulation of TH

In 1973, we proposed that cAMP mediates the increase in the biosynthesis of medullary TH elicited transsynaptically (Costa and Guidotti, 1973). Successive work has supported a crucial role of this second messenger in mediating the increase in the synthesis of TH elicited by cholinergic receptor activation (Guidotti and Costa, 1974a,b; Guidotti et al., 1975b; Costa and Guidotti, 1973; Costa et al., 1974a, 1975c,d). Since high doses of corticotropin can increase the cAMP content of the cortex and medulla (see Table II), it was suggested that the increase in medullary cAMP observed during a number of stresses which induce TH

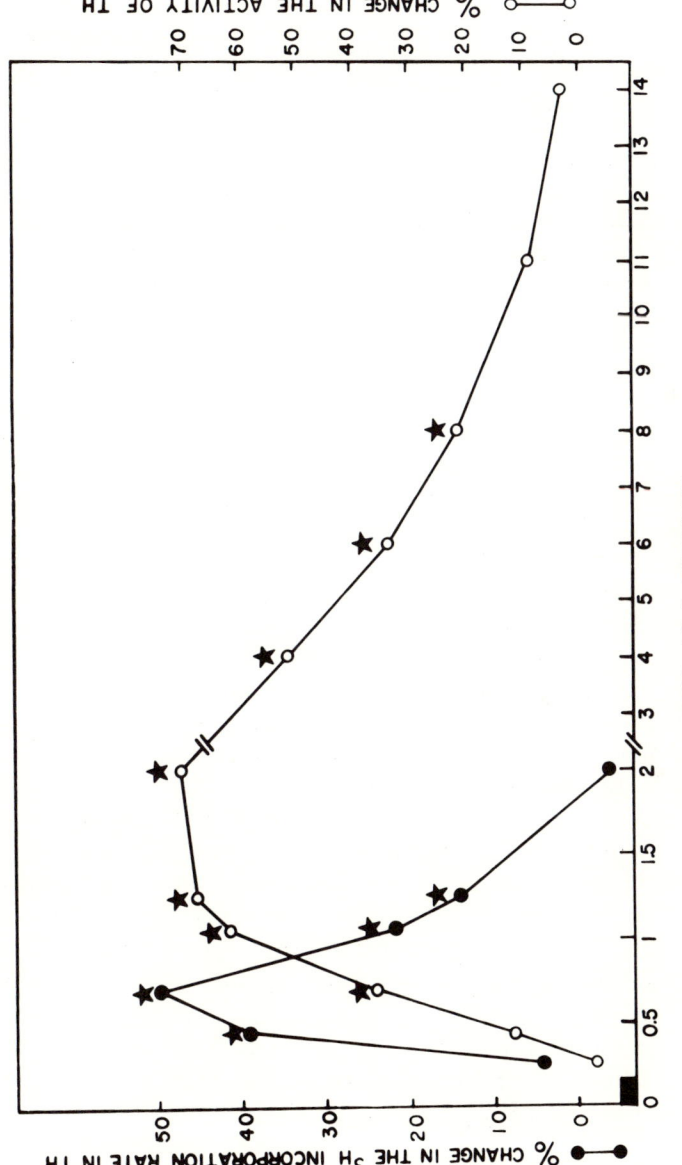

Fig. 1. Incorporation of ³H into immunochromatographically purified TH (90 min pulses at various times after the stimulus) and TH activity after the rats were kept at 0°C for 4 hr. (From Chuang and Costa, 1976, with permission.)

TABLE I

Selective Inhibition by Dexamethasone of the Increase of Cortical cAMP Content Elicited by Reserpine [a]

| | cAMP content (pmole/mg protein) | |
	Adrenal medulla	Adrenal cortex
Saline	28	10
Reserpine	75	110
Dexamethasone + reserpine	95	14

[a] Dexamethasone (0.2 μmole/kg ip) was injected 120 min before reserpine. Reserpine (16 μmole/kg ip) was injected 30 min (cortical cAMP) or 60 min (medullary cAMP) before killing the cats.

was due to an action of ACTH rather than acetylcholine on adrenal medulla (Thoenen and Otten, 1975). Data reported in another publication (Costa *et al.*, 1975d) and the experiments reported in Table I strongly suggest that the regulation of cAMP in adrenal medulla can be differentiated from the process that regulates cAMP in adrenal cortex (Costa *et al.*, 1975b).

The correlation between the early increase of cAMP content in medulla and the delayed increase of TH activity elicited by various stimuli is very convincing if comparison is made using, as a reference, an increase of the cAMP lasting for about 1 hr or longer (Table II). To some investigators it was not immediately apparent why the cAMP content had to be increased for 1 hr in order to trigger the TH induction (Thoenen and Otten, 1975). Now that we know that an activated cytosol protein kinase must be translocated from cytosol to the nucleus to increase mRNA synthesis, we can appreciate why the cAMP must increase for at least 1 hr in order to trigger the TH induction (Costa *et al.*, 1975d; Guidotti *et al.*, 1976). In fact, unless the protein kinase remains dissociated long enough it cannot be transported to the nucleus. This transport appears to depend on a process that is inhibited by colchicine (Kumakura, unpublished observations) and by a nuclear uptake (Chuang *et al.*, 1977).

E. Activation of cAMP-Dependent Protein Kinase as an Intermediate Step in the Transsynaptic Induction of TH

In 1968, Dr. Edwin Krebs and his colleagues (Krebs, 1972) made the important discovery that a cAMP-dependent protein kinase was present in skeletal muscle; moreover, they presented evidence that the effects of

TABLE II

Research between cAMP Content, Increase in Protein Kinase Activation Index, and Tyrosine TH Activity in Rat Adrenal Medulla

| Stimulus [a] | cAMP (pmole/mg) protein | | Kinase activation index at 1.5 hr [c] | TH (nmole/hr per gland) at 24 hr |
	0.5 hr	1 hr		
Carbamylcholine				
(3.2 μmole/kg ip)	280 ± 25	34 ± 8	0.18 ± 0.12	5 ± 0.5
(9.2 μmole/kg ip)	280 ± 35 [b]	100 ± 9 [b]	0.42 ± 0.05 [b]	11 ± 1.0 [b]
Reserpine				
(16 μmole/kg ip)	145 ± 12 [b]	70 ± 10 [b]	0.59 ± 0.03 [b]	10 ± 0.5 [b]
Exposure to 4° (2 hr)	190 ± 15 [b]	175 ± 20 [b]	0.48 ± 0.04 [b]	8.2 ± 0.8 [b]
Aminophylline				
(200 μmole/kg ip)	375 ± 40 [b]	350 ± 25 [b]	0.45 ± 0.04 [b]	9.2 ± 1.2 [b]
Corticotropin				
(1 IU/kg iv)	225 ± 18 [b]	38 ± 7	0.17 ± 0.005	6 ± 0.4
Dopamine				
(50 μmole/kg sc)	80 ± 7 [b]	32 ± 7	0.22 ± 0.03	4.8 ± 0.5
Propranolol				
(40 μmole/kg ip)	100 ± 6 [b]	25 ± 5	0.20 ± 0.01	5.5 ± 0.6

[a] ip, intraperitoneally; iv, intravenously; sc, subcutaneously. Corticotropin = ACTH.

[b] $p < .05$ when compared to saline-treated rats ($n = 5$).

[c] The kinase activation index is the ratio of the activity in 20,000g supernatant in the absence and presence of cAMP (0.7 μM). In all experiments, the phosphate acceptor was a calf thymus mixture of histones (300 μg/ml). Each point is the mean $\pm$ S.E. of five experiments. The concentration of cAMP in saline-treated rats was 28 ± 2 pmole/mg of protein; the kinase activation index was 0.18 ± 0.101; and the monooxygenase activity was 5 ± 5.0 nmole/hr per gland.

cAMP in regulating glycogen breakdown in skeletal muscle were mediated through the activation of a specific protein kinase by cAMP (Walsh *et al.*, 1970). Since cAMP-dependent protein kinases were found in a wide variety of animal tissues, the hypothesis was proposed that the diverse effects of cAMP in various tissues are mediated by activating specific protein kinases (Walsh *et al.*, 1970). The appalling aspect of this hypothesis was that it provided a mechanism by which a simple molecule like cAMP could regulate diversified physiological mechanisms, ranging from ion fluxes through cell membranes to glucose utilization and RNA transcription. These diversified actions mediated by cAMP could be explained by the specificity of the properties that the various protein kinase substrates acquire following phosphorylation. The cAMP-dependent protein kinase has the accepted subunit structure R_2C_2, where the R and C subunits are dissimilar (for review, see Nimmo and Cohen, 1977). In the absence of cAMP, the holoenzyme complex is inactive; when cAMP is added, the binding of cAMP to the regulatory receptor subunit results in a dissociation and consequent activation of the free catalytic subunits. Reconstitution of the whole enzyme complex of regulatory and catalytic subunit reconstitutes the cAMP dependence. The equilibrium expression is

$$R_2C_2 + 2 \text{ cAMP} \rightleftharpoons (R \text{ cAMP})_2 + 2 \text{ C}$$

The molecular weight of the tetramer ranges from 1.5 to 1.7×10^5. The molecular weight of the receptor dimer ranges from 4.2 to 5.5×10^4 and the catalytic subunit from 3.8 to 4.2×10^4. The holoenzyme has an isoelectic point of pH 5.1; the regulatory subunits have an isoelectric point of pH 4.5; the catalytic subunit range from pH 6.7 to 8.5. There are two types of cAMP-dependent protein kinases that can be separated by DEAE-cellulose chromatography in an NaCl gradient (Corbin and Keely, 1977; Corbin *et al.*, 1975).

The type I cAMP-dependent protein kinase is eluted with less than 0.1 M NaCl; and the type II is eluted at 0.15 to 0.2 M NaCl. Type I dissociates rapidly in the presence of histone or 0.5 M NaCl and reassociates slowly after removal of cAMP, which suggests that the R and C subunits of type I are held together by weaker forces than those of the type II enzyme. The type II enzyme undergoes phosphorylation with incorporation of 2 moles/PO_4^{-3} per receptor dimer of protein kinase. Phosphorylation enhances dissociation by cAMP and slows down reassociation. Type II holoenzyme is more slowly dissociated into subunits by histone and 0.5 M NaCl, and reassociates rapidly on cAMP removal, which suggests tighter attractive forces between the subunits. It is currently believed that type I and type II protein kinase are the two functional forms of the enzyme; however, a great deal of indirect evidence indicates that each of the two types of enzymes includes important subdivisions, which are not thoroughly understood.

The adrenal medulla of rats contains types I and II (Costa *et al.*, 1978) cAMP-dependent protein kinases which are activated by the stimulation of nicotinic receptors (Guidotti *et al.*, 1975b). Both enzyme forms are almost exclusively located in cytosol, where a cAMP-independent protein kinase is also located. Whereas medullary cytosol contains a high proportion of histone kinase, the nucleus contains two molecular forms that phosphorylate acidic proteins, in addition to high-molecular-weight histone kinase. To increase the reliability of the measurements of cAMP content, as an index of the participation of the second messenger in the mediation of a response, together with these values, we have reported in Table II the index of protein kinase activation. It is clear that the results of the measurement of cAMP content at 30 min fail to establish any correlation between the increase in cAMP content, the activation of cAMP-dependent protein kinase, and the delayed induction of TH. A positive correlation appears to exist if one considers the cAMP measurements at 1 hr (Table II) (Guidotti *et al.*, 1975b; Costa *et al.*, 1975a,c, 1976). Then it is possible to show that a specific metabolic signal lasting 1 hr can activate protein kinase; this activation participates in eliciting a trophic response in the medulla which peaks 24 hr later and lasts several days. Activation of protein kinase can occur in association with the changes in the total amount of enzyme present. In order to elaborate whether or not, during the transsynaptic activation of protein kinase, the total amount of cytosol enzyme changed, we measured, at various times after reserpine (16 moles/kg ip), the protein kinase activity in the pellet and cytosol of the adrenal medulla (Fig. 2). The data show that the protein kinase activity of the pellet increases within a few hours following the reserpine injection, whereas, the cytosol activity decreases with a time course identical to the increase in the activity of the pellet. Both changes reach a peak in about 8 hr and their value returns to basal level in about 24 hr (Kurosawa *et al.*, 1976a). Following the increase of medullary cAMP content, there is a change in the subcellular distribution of the cAMP-dependent protein kinase. Since the total enzyme activity (pellet + cytosol) was not changed at various times after reserpine, we surmised that the changes shown in Fig. 2 were due to a relocation of the enzyme (Costa *et al.*, 1976; Kurosawa *et al.*, 1976). This suggestion has prompted a series of questions.

1. Are both types of cytosol protein kinases involved in the translocation?

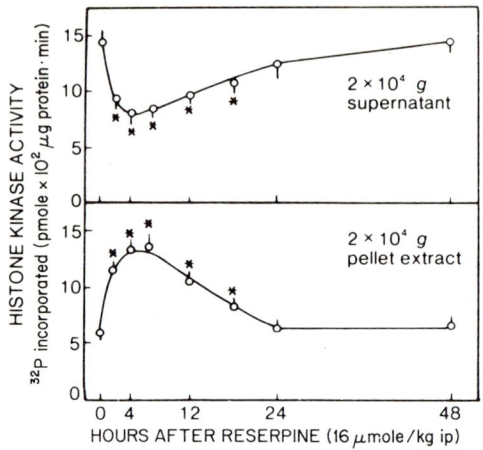

Fig. 2. Time course of histone kinase activity in the 20,000g supernatant and pellet extract of adrenal medulla homogenate from reserpine-injected rats. Six pairs of animals were sacrificed at various times after the administration of 16 μmole/kg ip of reserpine. The 20,000g supernatant of adrenal medulla homogenate was prepared as described in Costa *et al.* (1976). The pellet was extracted with 120 μl of 0.5 *M* NaCl, 10 m*M* potassium phosphate buffer (pH 6.5), 10 m*M* EDTA, 5 m*M* aminophylline, 0.2% Triton X-100. The assay was performed in the presence of 0.7 μmole of cAMP and Triton mixture. Each values is the mean S.E. of six determinations. (From Costa *et al.,* 1976. with permission.)

2. Is the nucleus a territory for enzyme relocation?

3. What is the role of nuclear protein phosphorylation in transcription?

During the transsynaptic induction of TH, types I and II cAMP-dependent protein kinases are activated (Guidotti and Costa, 1977). In 2–3 hr after the stimulus application, the cytosol content of type I is decreased (Costa *et al.,* 1978) and remains low for about 24 hr (Kurosawa *et al.,* 1976b). This decrease is not due to enzyme activation because type II protein kinase is activated for as long as the cAMP content remains elevated, but its content remains unchanged. Investigation of the precise location of the protein kinase translocated into the pellet reveals that the protein kinase activity of the nucleus is increased. By using specific inhibitors of cAMP-dependent protein kinase and performing enzyme recombination experiments, it was shown that the increase was due to the uptake into the nucleus of catalytic subunits of cytosol cAMP-dependent protein kinase (Costa *et al.,* 1976; Kurosawa *et al.,* 1976b). Moreover, it was shown that this newly taken up enzyme increased the phosphorylation of the endogenous nuclear protein. This finding is implemented by recent experiments (Kumakura *et al.*, 1979) on primary cultures of chromaffin cells prepared according to Waymire *et al.* (1977).

F. Nuclear Translocation of Cytosol Protein Kinase and the Transsynaptic Induction of TH in Adrenal Medulla

The nucleus of chromaffin cells contains various molecular forms of protein kinases. These can be characterized according to molecular size, substrate specificity, mobility in DEAE-50 cellulose column, susceptibility to cAMP activation, and to the inhibition by the specific endogenous protein inhibitor (Hollenbeck *et al.*, 1978; Chuang *et al.*, 1977). These studies have revealed that cAMP-dependent protein kinase is not present in the nuclei. However, when the nuclei of chromaffin cells were incubated *in vitro* with cAMP-dependent protein kinase (Chuang *et al.*, 1977) or when the cytosol protein kinase was activated for a protracted time period (Costa *et al.*, 1976; Kurosawa *et al.*, 1976b), there was an uptake of the enzyme into the nucleus. This uptake process was followed by a progressive modification of the properties of the newly taken up catalytic subunit of protein kinase. These changes occur gradually following the enzyme uptake into the nucleus. Immediately following this uptake, the specific affinity for basic histone and other basic substrates is lost. The cAMP-dependent protein kinase from cytosol has a limited affinity for acidic protein, but, following its uptake into the nucleus, it acquires a better affinity for casein. The mechanism for such a change is presently being studied. After its uptake the catalytic subunit of cAMP-dependent protein kinase from cytosol also loses the capability of being inhibited by the specific endogenous protein inhibitor; later it even loses the capability of being regulated by the regulatory subunits and thereby becomes a cAMP-independent enzyme. Since in basal conditions the amount of nuclear protein kinase activity that can be inhibited by the addition of regulatory subunits is negligible, we can infer that the rate of catalytic subunit translocation is rather slow. We cannot decide whether translocation of cytosol protein kinase into the nucleus is a continuous, slow process that increases dramatically when the nuclear transcription process requires modification, such as during transsynaptic induction, or if it is a discontinuous process that occurs only in certain contingencies. In certain conditions, we have detected regulatory subunits of cAMP-dependent protein kinase that have translocated from cytosol to the nucleus of chromaffin cells (Chuang *et al.*, 1977). The relative proportion of the two proteins is not stoichiometrical; once they reach the nucleus, the two proteins must occupy separate compartments, otherwise the protein kinase activity could not be expressed in the absence of cAMP. Perhaps regulatory and catalytic units that translocate simultaneously function as separate entities. It is possible that when a regulatory subunit reaches a catalytic subunit located in a certain metabolic compartment of the nucleus, it binds to it, and thereby prevents the expression of the enzyme activity. Thus, by alternating binding of regulatory or catalytic units or both, specific instructions for the phosphorylation of specific nuclear protein reach the nucleus. Since chromatin phosphorylation increases the rate of transcription, this modulation of chromatin phosphorylation by translocation of cytosol protein kinase is an important regulatory process (Chuang *et al.,* 1976). Translocation is probably a code of communication between receptors in cell membranes and nuclei. The keys to the existence of such a code are the detection of translocation in association with an increase in translation (Costa *et al.,* 1975d, 1976; Kurosawa *et al.,* 1976b), and the detection of a specific uptake process for the passage of these proteins from cytoplasm to specific nucleoplasmic sites, where the enzyme taken up can express its activity on endogenous substrates (Chuang *et al.,* 1977).

The catalytic subunits taken up by the nucleus form strong ionic bonds with chromatin protein (Chuang *et al.,* 1977; Costa *et al.,* 1974b). This ionic binding persists at a very high salt concentration (Chuang *et al.,* 1977; Costa *et al.,* 1974b). These findings have suggested to us that the newly taken up catalytic subunits (by phosphorylating specific proteins) can regulate RNA transcription, as we have shown to occur with chromatin *in vitro* (Chuang *et al.,* 1976). But equally important for such regulation may be the uptake of regulatory subunits that, either by binding to previously taken up catalytic subunits or by phosphorylating sites that should not be phosphorylated, limit the function of the newly taken up catalytic subunits. We currently believe that translocation of catalytic and regulatory subunits of cyclic AMP-dependent protein kinase may be a mechanism which could explain specific regulation of RNA translation by transsynaptic stimuli.

III. CONCLUSIONS

In our attempts to recognize the participation of various molecular events in the regulation of circulatory function, we have described a transsynaptic mechanism which exerts long-term effects on postsynaptic cells. However, the system that we have described lacks flexibility in the modulation of the response duration. In fact, it does not depend only on the nature of the communication process but also on the $T_{1/2}$ of the protein that is being modulated. When the protein is TH, which has a long $T_{1/2}$ (see Fig. 1), the duration of the regulatory process is long-lasting. We have proposed that translocation of regulatory and catalytic subunits of cAMP-dependent protein kinase may be a code in the communication of receptors located in the cell membrane and in the cell nucleus.

REFERENCES

Axelrod, J. (1971). Noradrenaline: fate and control of its biosynthesis. *Science* **173,** 598–606.

Bromstrom, C. D., Huang, T.-C., Breckenridge, B. McL., and Wolff, D. J. (1975). Identification of a calcium-binding protein as a calcium dependent regulator of brain adenylate cyclase. *Proc. Natl. Acad. Sci. U.S.A.* **72,** 64–68.

Cheung, W. Y., Lin, Y. M., Liu, Y. P., and Smoake, J. A. (1975). Regulation of bovine brain cyclic 3′, 5′-nucleotide phosphodiesterase by its protein activator. *In* "Cyclic Nucleotides in Disease" (B. Weiss, ed.), pp. 321–350. Univ. Park Press, Baltimore, Maryland.

Chuang, D. M., and Costa, E. (1974). Biosynthesis of tyrosine hydroxylase in rat adrenal medulla after exposure to cold. *Proc. Natl. Acad. Sci. U.S.A.* **71,** 4570–4574.

Chuang, D. M., and Costa, E. (1976). Transsynaptic regulation of ribonucleic acid biosynthesis in rat adrenal medulla. *Mol. Pharmacol.* **12,** 514–518.

Chuang, D. M., Zsilla, G., and Costa, E. (1975). Turnover rate of tyrosine hydroxylase during transsynaptic induction. *Mol. Pharmacol.* **11,** 784–794.

Chuang, D. M., Hollenbeck, R., and Costa, E. (1976). Enhanced template activity in chromatin from adrenal medulla after phosphorylation of chromosomal proteins *Science* **193,** 60–62.

Chuang, D. M., Hollenbeck, R. A., and Costa, E. (1977). Protein phosphorylation in nuclei of adrenal medulla incubated with cyclic adenosine 3′:5′-monophosphate-dependent protein kinase. *J. Biol. Chem.* **252,** 8365–8373.

Corbin, J. D., and Keely, S. L. (1977). Characterization and regulation of heart adenosine 3′:5′-monophosphate-dependent protein kinase isozymes. *J. Biol. Chem.* **252,** 910–918.

Corbin, J. D., Keely, S. L., and Park, C. R. (1975). The distribution and dissociation of cyclic adenosine 3′:5′-monophosphate-dependent protein kinases in adipose, cardiac, and other tissues. *J. Biol. Chem.* **250,** 218–225.

Costa, E., and Guidotti, A. (1973). The role of 3′, 5′-cyclic adenosine monophosphate in the regulation of adrenal medullary function. *In* "New Concepts in Neurotransmitter Regulation" (A. J. Mandell, ed.), pp. 135–152. Plenum, New York.

Costa, E., Guidotti, A., and Hanbauer, I. (1974a). Do cyclic nucleotides promote the transsynaptic induction of tyrosine hydroxylase *Life Sci.* **14,** 1169–1188.

Costa, E., Guidotti, A., and Zivkovic, B. (1974b). Short- and long-term regulation of tyrosine hydroxylase. *In* "Neuropsychopharmacology of Monoamines and Their Regulatory Enzymes" (E. Usdin, ed.), Advances in Biochemical Psychopharmacology, Vol. 12, pp. 161–175. Raven, New York.

Costa, E., Chuang, D. M., Guidotti, A., and Uzunov, P. (1975a). Cyclic 3′, 5′ adenosine monophosphate dependent molecular mechanisms in the transsynaptic induction of tyrosine hydroxylase in rat adrenal medulla. In "Chemical Tools in Catecholamine Research II" (O. Almgren, A. Carlsson, and J. Engel, eds.), pp. 283–292. North-Holland Publ., Amsterdam.

Costa, E., Guidotti, A., and Hanbauer, I. (1975b). Comment on the paper: "Lack of correlation between rate of increase in cAMP and subsequent induction of tyrosine hydroxylase in sympathetic ganglia and adrenal medulla." In "Neuropsychopharmacology" (J. R. Boissier, H. Hippius, and P. Pichot, eds.), pp. 952–955. Excerpta Med., Found., Amsterdam.

Costa, E., Guidotti, A., and Hanbauer, I. (1975c). Cyclic nucleotides and trophism of secretory cells: Study of adrenal medulla. In "Cyclic Nucleotides in Disease" (B. Weiss, ed.), pp. 167–186. Univ. Park Press, Baltimore, Maryland.

Costa, E., Guidotti, A., and Kurosawa, A. (1975d). Evidence for a role of protein kinase activation and translocation in the transsynaptic control of tyrosine hydroxylase biosynthesis. In "Biological Membranes—Neurochemistry" (Y. Raoul, ed.), Vol. 41, pp. 137–149. North-Holland Publ., Amsterdam.

Costa, E., Kurosawa, A., and Guidotti, A. (1976). Activation and nuclear translocation of protein kinase during transsynaptic induction of tyrosine 3-monooxygenase. Proc. Natl. Acad. Sci. U.S.A. 73, 1058–1062.

Costa, E., Chuang, D. M., Guidotti, A., and Hollenbeck, R. (1978). Control of nuclear function in chromaffin cells by persistent activation of nicotinic receptors. In "Cholinergic Mechanisms and Psychopharmacology" (D. J. Jenden, ed.), pp. 267–284. Plenum, New York.

Di Giulio, A. M., Yang, H.-Y. T., Lutold, B., Fratta, W., Hong, J., and Costa, E. (1978). Characterization of enkephalin-like material extracted from sympathetic ganglia. Neuropharmacology 17, 989–992.

Gopinath, R. M., and Vincenzi, F. F. (1977). Phosphodiesterase protein activator mimics red blood cell cytoplasmic activator of (Ca⁺⁺, Mg⁺⁺) ATPase. Biochem. Biophys. Res. Commun. 77, 1203–1209.

Guidotti, A., and Costa, E. (1973). Involvement of adenosine 3′, 5′ -monophosphate in the activation of tyrosine hydroxylase elicited by drugs. Science 179, 902–904.

Guidotti, A., and Costa, E. (1974a). A role for nicotinic receptors in the regulation of the adenylate cyclase of adrenal medulla. J. Pharmacol. Exp. Ther. 189, 665–675.

Guidotti, A., and Costa, E. (1974b). Association between increase in cyclic AMP and subsequent induction of tyrosine hydroxylase in rat adrenal medulla. Naunyn-Schmiedeberg's Arch. Pharmacol. 282, 217–221.

Guidotti, A., and Costa, E. (1977). Transsynaptic regulation of tyrosine 3-mono-oxy-genase biosynthesis in rat adrenal medulla. Biochem. Pharmacol. 26, 817–823.

Guidotti, A., Mao, C. C., and Costa, E. (1973). Transsynaptic regulation of tyrosine hydroxylase in adrenal medulla: Possible role of cyclic nucleotides. In "Frontiers in Catecholamine Research" (E. Usdin and S. H. Snyder, eds.), pp. 231–236. Pergamon, Oxford.

Guidotti, A., Hanbauer, I., and Costa, E. (1975a). Role of cyclic nucleotides in the induction of tyrosine hydroxylase. In "Advances in Cyclic Nucleotide Research, Vol. 5 " (G. I. Drummond, P. Greenwood, and G. A. Robinson, eds.), pp. 619–639. Raven Press, New York.

Guidotti, A., Kurosawa, A., Chuang, D. M., and Costa, E. (1975b). Protein kinase activation as an early event in the transsynaptic induction of tyrosine 3-monoxy-genase in adrenal medulla. Proc. Natl. Acad. Sci. U.S.A. 72, 1152–1156.

Guidotti, A., Kurosawa, A., and Costa, E. (1976). Association between the increase of cAMP content and the transsynaptic induction of tyrosine hydroxylase in rat adrenal medulla. *Naunyn-Schmiedberg's Arch. Pharmacol.* **295**, 135–140.

Hanbauer, I., and Guidotti, A. (1975). Further evidence for a cAMP dependent regulation of tyrosine-3-monoxygenase induction in adrenal medulla. *Naunyn-Schmeideberg's Arch. Pharmacol.* **287**, 213–217.

Hanbauer, I., Guidotti, A., and Costa, E. (1975). Involvement of cyclic nucleotides in the long term induction of tyrosine hydroxylase. *In* "Neuropsychopharmacology" (J. R. Boissier, H. Hippius, and P. Pichot, eds.), pp. 932–941. Excerpta Med. Found., Amsterdam.

Hollenbeck, R. A., Chuang, D. M., and Costa, E. (1978). Characterization of protein kinases from adrenal medulla. A study of cytosol and nuclear enzymes. *Neurochem. Res.* **3**, 49–67.

Joh, T. H., Geghman, C., and Reis, D. (1973). Immunochemical demonstration of increased accumulation of tyrosine hydroxylase protein in sympathetic ganglia and adrenal medulla elicited by reserpine. *Proc. Natl. Acad. Sci. U.S.A.* **70**, 2767–2771.

Klee, C. B. (1977). Conformational transition accompanying the binding of Ca++ to the protein activator of 3', 5'-cyclic adenosine monophosphate phosphodiesterase. *Biochemistry* **16**, 1017–1024.

Krebs, E. G. (1972). Protein kinases. *In* "Current Topics in Cellular Regulation" (B. L. Horecker and E. R. Stadtman, eds.) Vol. 5, pp. 99–133. Academic Press, New York.

Kumakura, K., Guidotti, A., and Costa, E. (1978). Effect of colchicine on cAMP-mediated induction of tyrosine hydroxylase (TH) in cultured bovine adrenal chromaffin cells. *Pharmacologist* **20**, 218.

Kumakara, K., Guidotti, A., and Costa, E. (1979). Primary cultures of chromaffin cells: Molecular mechanisms for the induction of tyrosine hydroxylase mediated by 8-Br-cyclic AMP. *Mol. Pharmacol.* **16**, 865–876.

Kurosawa, A., Guidotti, A., and Costa, E. (1976a). Induction of tyrosine 3-monooxygenase elicited by carbamylcholine in intact and denervated adrenal medulla: Role of protein kinase activation and translocation. *Mol. Pharmacol.* **12**, 420–432.

Kurosawa, A., Guidotti, A., and Costa, E. (1976b). Induction of tyrosine 3-monooxygenase in adrenal medulla: Role of protein kinase activation and translocation. *Science* **193**, 691–693.

Nimmo, H. G., and Cohen, P. (1977). Hormonal control of protein phosphorylation. *In* "Advances in Cyclic Nucleotide Research, Vol. 8." (P. Greengard and G. A. Robinson, eds.), pp. 145–266. Raven Press, New York.

Otten, U., Mueller, R. A. Oesch, F., and Thoenen, H. (1974a). Location of an isoproterenol-responsive cyclic AMP pool in adrenergic nerve cell bodies and its relationship to tyrosine 3-mono oxygenase induction. *Proc. Natl. Acad. Sci. U.S.A.* **71**, 2217–2221.

Otten, U., Mueller, R. A., and Thoenen, H. (1974b). Evidence against a causal relationship between increase in cAMP and induction of tyrosine hydroxylase in the rat adrenal medulla. *Naunyn-Schmiedeberg's Arch. Pharmacol.* **285**, 233–242.

Robison, G. A., Butcher, R. W., and Sutherland, E. W. (1971). "Cyclic AMP." Academic Press, New York.

Schneider, A. S., Herz, R., and Rosenheck, K. (1977). Stimulus-secretion coupling in chromaffin cells isolated from bovine adrenal medulla. *Proc. Natl. Acad. Sci. U.S.A.* **74**, 5036–5040.

Sutherland, E. W., and Rall, T. W. (1960). The relation of adenosine-3', 5'-phosphate and phosphorylase to the actions of catecholamines and other hormones. *Pharmacol. Rev.* **12**, 265–299.

Thoenen, H., and Otten, U. (1975). Cyclic nucleotides and transsynaptic enzyme induction: Lack of correlation between initial cAMP increase, changes in cAMP/ cGMP ratio and subsequent induction of tyrosine hydroxylase in the adrenal medulla. *In* "Chemical Tools in Catecholamine Research II" (O. Almgren, A. Carlsson, and J. Engel, eds.), pp. 275–282. North-Holland Publ., Amsterdam.

Thoenen, H., Mueller, R. A., and Axelrod, J. (1969a). Transsynaptic induction of adrenal tyrosine hydroxylase. *J. Pharmacol. Exp. Ther.* **169,** 249–254.

Thoenen, H., Mueller, R. A., and Axelrod, J. (1969b). Increased tyrosine hydroxylase activity after drug-induced alteration of sympathetic transmission. *Nature (London)* **221,** 1264–1270.

Thoenen, H., Otten, U., and Oesch, F. (1973). Transsynaptic regulation of tyrosine hydroxylase. *In* "Frontiers in Catecholamine Research" (E. Usdin and S. H. Snyder, eds.), pp. 179–185. Pergamon, Oxford.

Walsh, D. A., Krebs, E. G., Reimann, E. M., Brostrom, M. A., Corbin, J. D., Hickenbottom, J. P., Soderling, T. R., and Perkins, J. P. (1970). The receptor protein for cyclic AMP in the control of glycogenolysis. *In* "Role of Cyclic AMP in Cell Function" (P. Greengard and E. Costa, eds.), Advances in Biochemical Psychopharmacology, Vol. 3, pp. 265–285. Raven, New York.

Waymire, J. C., Waymire, K. G., Boehme, R., Noritake, D., and Wardell, J. (1977). Regulation of tyrosine hydroxylase by cyclic 3′, 5-′adenosine monophosphate in cultured neuroblastoma and cultured dissociated bovine adrenal chromaffin cells. *In* "Structure and Function of Monoamine Enzymes" (E. Usdin, N. Weiner, and M. Youdim, eds.), pp. 327–363. Dekker, New York.

Weiss, B., and Costa, E. (1967). Adenyl cyclase activity in rat pineal gland: Effects of chronic denervation and norepinephrine. *Science* **156,** 1750–1752.

6

Neural Control of the
Circulation during
Hypoxia

John A. Krasney and Raymond C. Koehler

I. INTRODUCTION

Systemic hypoxia may be induced accidentally or experimentally by interfering with the passage of oxygen from the air into the blood in the lungs. This could occur as a result of a mechanical obstruction of the respiratory passages, alterations of the pulmonary circulation where there is admixture of arterial and venous blood, or as a consequence of inhalation of air containing oxygen at subnormal pressure (Lambertsen, 1961). The latter type of hypoxia is characterized by a reduction in blood oxygen content as well as oxygen tension. This is termed by some as arterial hypoxia or hypoxic hypoxia (Korner, 1959).

Primary tissue hypoxia may be induced by substances which poison cellular respiratory enzyme systems, such as cyanide or hydrogen sulfide (Anitchkov and Belen'kii, 1963; Korner, 1959). In the case of cyanide, there is no reduction in arterial oxygen content and arterial oxygen tension is not lowered.

The respiratory and cardiovascular responses to arterial hypoxia and

NEURAL CONTROL OF CIRCULATION

to primary tissue hypoxia are similar, and generally it is believed that the neural control mechanisms causing these responses are the same for both types (Comroe and Mortimer, 1964). Hyperventilation is elicited by systemic hypoxia, and this in turn produces hypocapnia and respiratory alkalosis as a consequence of the increased pulmonary ventilation. Reduction of P_{O_2} in tissues locally causes vasodilation and reduced vascular resistance in the coronary and cerebral beds, and in skeletal muscle (Korner, 1959). The mean arterial blood pressure increases; this is partly due to peripheral vasoconstrictor nerve discharge being reflexly derived from hypoxemic stimulation of the peripheral chemoreceptors, and partly due to an increase in cardiac output. The elevated arterial pressure may act in concert with local variations in vascular resistance to produce a compensatory regional redistribution of blood flow so as to maintain an adequate oxygen supply to the central nervous system (Anitchkov and Belen'kii, 1963).

It has been known for some time that the elevation of the cardiac output during hypoxia is produced mainly by an increase in the heart rate and to a lesser degree by an increase in stroke volume (Korner, 1959). These circulatory adjustments occur in concert with an increased respiratory tidal volume and frequency. It should be emphasized that the sensitivity of the circulatory control mechanisms to hypoxia exceeds that of the respiratory mechanisms because the first observed alteration in response to hypoxia is cardiac acceleration, which occurs at arterial P_{O_2} levels well above those at which increased respiratory activity is observed (Comroe, 1965).

It is evident that the mechanisms concerned with cardiovascular regulation during systemic hypoxia have been studied intensively. However, the factors involved in hypoxic neural control of the circulation remain controversial and are not well understood. The confusion that is extant in the literature concerning cardiovascular regulation is largely due to differences in experimental protocol, the type and severity of the hypoxic exposure, and the complicating influences of anesthesia. Therefore, this review will be limited to an analysis of neural circulatory control, and, in particular, to the control of cardiac dynamics as it occurs during acute and progressive arterial hypoxia in a particular animal model, insofar as is possible, i.e., the conscious, chronically instrumented dog.

II. BACKGROUND

The physiological basis for the cardiac acceleration of hypoxia and the increment in cardiac output was not considered to be a problem until the studies of Bernthal *et al.* (1951). Prior to that time, it had generally been assumed (Korner, 1959) that hypoxic stimulation of the carotid body chemoreceptors was responsible for the production of tachycardia. Bernthal *et al.* (1951) surgically isolated and perfused the carotid bodies of a dog, either directly from a donor dog or by means of a perfusion pump. The carotid bodies of the recipient dog were perfused with hypoxic blood, while the remainder of the animal was oxygenated. When the carotid bodies of spontaneously breathing dogs were made hypoxic, the heart rate either rose, remained constant, or decreased. In dogs under artificial ventilation, hypoxic stimulation of the carotid bodies produced a decrease in heart rate in most of the animals while in some, the heart rate remained constant. Bernthal *et al.* (1951) concluded that reflex influences from the carotid bodies were not concerned with production of the tachycardia of hypoxia, but, on the other hand, stimulation of these structures may actually evoke a slowing of the heart rate.

Daly and Scott (1964) produced hypoxia in dogs by ventilating them with 7–12% O_2 in N_2. This procedure elicited an elevation of cardiac output, as determined by dye dilution, an increase in heart rate, and a reduction in total peripheral resistance. The carotid bodies were isolated and perfused with blood from a tube attached to a cannula inserted in the dog's own femoral artery. Subsequently, the carotid bodies were perfused with oxygenated blood while the animal remained hypoxic. This procedure produced a rise in heart rate despite the fact that the preexisting heart rate was elevated. This change was accompanied by a further elevation of the cardiac output, by a reduction in respiratory minute volume, and by a further decrease in total peripheral resistance. When hypoxemic perfusion of the carotid bodies was reinstituted, these effects were reversed. Daly and Scott (1964) concluded that the increased heart rate during systemic hypoxia could not be attributed to effects produced by stimulation of the carotid bodies; in fact, these structures may produce effects which antagonize the rise in heart rate.

Downing *et al.* (1962) studied the cardiovascular changes produced by stimulation of vascularly isolated carotid bodies. They induced systemic hypoxia in control experiments and observed tachycardia accompanied by elevated cardiac output. In contrast, perfusion of isolated carotid bodies with blood of low oxygen tension elicited a decrease in heart rate and a reduction of the cardiac output. Bilateral vagotomy reduced, but did not eliminate, the negative chronotropic action. Downing *et al.* (1962) did not observe a decrease in heart rate in response to carotid body stimulation after blockade of autonomic ganglia by hexamethonium. These results indicated that the decrease in heart rate observed during stimulation of the carotid bodies was partly due to increased vagal inhibition and partly due to a reduction in tonic activity of the cardioaccelerator nerves. It is apparent from studies such as these that the chemoreceptors of the carotid body do not contribute to the cardiac acceleration during systemic hypoxia.

Comroe and Mortimer (1964) concluded that stimulation of the aortic body chemoreceptors can account for the tachycardia of hypoxia. They bilaterally inserted long coiled catheters into the common carotid arteries in the midcervical region to delay the arrival of drugs, injected into the region of the aortic arch, to the carotid bodies. The drugs were introduced into the circulation through a catheter tip positioned in the aortic arch. The circulation time of drugs from the aortic arch to the carotid sinus region, via the coils, ranged from 15–75 sec. Comroe and Mortimer observed that a "typical'" response pattern to cyanide (a potent chemoreceptor stimulant) in the aortic arch consisted of hyperventilation, hypertension, and tachycardia, in the first 2 sec after injection; about 60 sec later, hyperventilation, bradycardia, and hypotension were observed. The authors considered the first response that occurred immediately after injection to be a result of aortic-body stimulation, but they considered the later response to be due to carotid-body stimulation. However, the "typical" response did not consistently occur. An atypical response such as cardiac slowing or no heart rate change was observed in 33 dogs on the initial aortic-body response, while the so-called typical responses occurred in 21 dogs. In view of these experimental results, it may be likely that the aortic bodies contribute in part to the tachycardia of systemic hypoxia, but other explanations are possible. The hypotensive response to carotid-body stimulation is contrary to the hypertensive response observed by others (Daly and Scott, 1960; Downing et al., 1962). The results may have been influenced by other receptors located in the vicinity of the aortic arch or, as suggested by Comroe and Mortimer (1964), the presence of heterogenous cell populations in the aortic bodies could account for the variations.

Daly and Scott (1963) postulated that activation of afferent neurons from pulmonary stretch receptors by the hyperventilation of hypoxia is in part responsible for the hypoxic cardiac responses. They noted that stimulation of isolated dog carotid bodies with hypoxic blood in spontaneously breathing animals caused either an increase, a decrease, or no change in heart rate. In contrast, stimulation of the carotid bodies of artificially ventilated dogs, dogs with denervated lungs, or dogs with constant arterial P_{CO_2} consistently caused a slowing of the heart rate. Daly and Scott (1963) pointed to the well-known observation that stimulation of the central end of the sectioned vagus nerve elicits tachycardia. They concluded that elimination of the hyperventilation and concomitant hypocapnia associated with carotid body stimulation unmasks the primary cardioinhibitory carotid body response.

Kontos *et al.* (1965a) extended the studies of Daly and Scott (1963) to dogs exposed to systemic hypoxia. Pulmonary stretch-receptor afferents were inactivated by ventilating the animal by means of a constant-stroke respirator, and by blocking respiratory efforts with decamethonium. They induced systemic hypoxia by ventilating the animal with 7.5% O_2 for a period of 10 min. Spontaneously breathing dogs showed increases in cardiac output, heart rate, and mean arterial blood pressure. Dogs under controlled ventilation, on the other hand, responded to systemic hypoxia with significant decreases in heart rate. Cardiac output was not altered, but mean arterial pressure increased. It was also found that prevention of hypocapnia by maintenance of constant arterial P_{CO_2} in spontaneously breathing dogs significantly diminished the tachycardia of hypoxia induced by ventilation with 7.5% O_2 in N_2. These results are in accord with the hypothesis of Daly and Scott (1963) who believe the tachycardia of systemic hypoxia is produced in part by activation of reflexes associated with increased respiratory activity. In order to further substantiate this point, Kontos *et al.* (1970) selectively inactivated the carotid-body chemoreceptors by close arterial injection of the acetic acid. When the dogs were made hypoxic during controlled ventilation, the characteristic hypoxic bradycardia occurred. However, after inactivation of the carotid bodies, hypoxia produced a tachycardia, even though the dogs were artifically ventilated. These latter observations suggest that additional mechanisms are involved in the genesis of the cardiac response to hypoxia. The cardioaccelerator response to hypoxia persists after denervation of the lungs (Daly and Scott, 1963) and after inactivation of the carotid and aortic bodies (Davenport *et al.*, 1947).

Sands and DeGraff (1925) studied the role of the vagus nerves in the efferent control of this cardiac response. They allowed dogs to rebreathe air from a spirometer that contained a soda–lime canister. The effects on heart rate of hypoxia induced in this manner were studied before and after vagotomy. A control dog showed a slow, steady increase in heart rate during rebreathing, until a maximum rate of 190 beats/min was reached at 50 min with the spirometer O_2 concentration at 10%. In a vagotomized dog, no cardiac acceleration was observed until an O_2 concentration of 11% was reached after 55 min. After 85 min with the spirometer O_2 concentration at 2%, a maximum heart rate of 180 beats/min was reached. Sands and DeGraff (1925) concluded that in less severe hypoxia, the rise in heart rate is primarily a result of a reduction in vagal tone; whereas in more severe hypoxia (less than 10% O_2 in inspired air), stimulation of sympathetic activity takes place. These experimental results lend support to the hypothesis of Comroe and Mortimer (1964) that the aortic bodies play a role in less severe hypoxia, but they tend to rule out the possibility of the aortic bodies having a major role in the response to more severe hypoxia.

Nahas *et al.* (1954) attempted to assess the role of the sympathetic nerves in the cardiac response to hypoxia. They ventilated intact spontaneously breathing dogs with 8% O_2 for 15 min and observed a 56% increase in cardiac output and a 24% increase in heart rate, above the control levels. Six dogs were subjected to bilateral thoracic sympathectomy. It was noted that this procedure reduced the magnitude of the cardiac output increase to 23%, while the heart rate rose only 16% during exposure to hypoxia. The authors concluded that the ability of the circulatory system to adapt to hypoxia is diminished after extirpation of the cardiac sympathetic nerves.

The effects of total cardiac denervation on the response to hypoxia were studied by Glick *et al.* (1964). The method of Cooper *et al.* (1961) was employed. This involves complete regional ablation of the cardiac nerves. Failure to show an accelerator response to a tyramine infusion was used as a criterion of a complete denervation. Conscious animals were ventilated with 8% O_2 for 15 min. It was observed that the heart rates and cardiac indices were not significantly greater than the control measurements during the early stages of hypoxia, but these parameters significantly increased during the later stages of hypoxia. Glick *et al.* (1964) concluded that dogs with denervated hearts were not at a disadvantage during hypoxia, with respect to cardiovascular reactivity. They suggested that metabolic or humoral factors leading to a change in pacemaker automaticity were of greater importance than the cardiac innervation, in the maintenance of the cardiac output in hypoxia.

Nahas *et al.* (1954) studied the role of the adrenal gland in hypoxia by subjecting five dogs to chronic bilateral adrenalectomy. These dogs were ventilated with 8% O_2 for a period of 3 min. None of the dogs lived more than 12 hr after the experiment. It was observed that none of the measured cardiovascular variables changed in response to hypoxia. This information was offered with reservations, however, since the control heart rates in the adrenalectomized dogs averaged 188 beats/min. This factor may have masked the appearance of a mechanism that had been functioning at its maximum prior to hypoxia.

Baugh *et al.* (1959) studied the effects of chronic adrenalectomy on the cardiac response to hypoxia. They found that 15 adrenalectomized dogs failed to show significant increases in heart rate or cardiac output in response to ventilation with 6% O_2 in N_2. They collected blood from intact hypoxic dogs and injected it into intact recipient dogs via a right atrial catheter. The total amount of blood infused amounted to 20% of the recipient dog's blood volume. The infusion of blood from hypoxic dogs led to significant increases in the heart rates of the recipients. In contrast, the infusion of blood obtained from hypoxic adrenalectomized dogs did not change the heart rates of the recipient animals. Baugh *et al.* concluded that since the elevated heart rates and cardiac outputs were abrogated by adrenalectomy and since an adrenomimetic substance was apparently liberated, no important role should be assigned to the cardioaccelerator nerves as mediators of the cardiac response to hypoxia.

Toyooka and Blake (1961), however, were unable to find any increase in urinary or circulatory catecholamines, as determined by bioassay in response to ventilation of dogs with 8–10% O_2 in N_2. They checked their bioassay method by releasing catecholamines with an intraarterial injection of carbamylcholine.

Chalmers *et al.* (1965) used adrenergic and ganglionic blocking agents to study the activity of the sympathetic nervous system during hypoxia in the rabbit. It was found that the ganglion-blocking agent, trimetaphan, reduced the magnitude of the hypertensive response to hypoxia. The α-adrenergic receptor-blocking agent, dibenzyline, allowed a fall in arterial blood pressure in response to hypoxia. Finally, propranolol, an adrenergic β-receptor-blocking agent, unmasked a greater pressor response to hypoxia. Chalmers *et al.* deduced, from these observations, that sympathetic discharge occurs in hypoxia and that the net blood pressure effect is a result of the relative degree of α- and β-receptor stimulation taking place. The cardiac chronotropic response to hypoxia was also studied; however, the rabbit is a particularly vagotonic animal (Gesell and Hertzman, 1928) and systemic hypoxia actually causes a chemoreceptor-mediated, vagal-dependent bradycardia. Chalmers *et al.* (1965) observed a consistent reduction in heart rate during hypoxia with or without the influence of adrenergic blocking agents.

Krasney (1967) evaluated the comparative importance of the efferent neural and humoral components of the cardioaccelerator response to hypoxia in dogs anesthetized with chloralose. In contrast to the previously cited experiments, where hypoxia in the dog under controlled ventilation elicited a bradycardia, Krasney's dogs had lower control heart rates due to the morphine–chloralose anesthesia, and actually showed a tachycardia during hypoxia when ventilation was controlled. These cardioaccelerator responses to mild hypoxia were partially prevented by bilateral vagotomy. On the other hand, cardioaccelerator responses to a more severe oxygen lack or to cyanide in animals under the same experimental conditions, were not significantly reduced by vagotomy. This result indicates that a part of the accelerator response to mild hypoxia is related to inhibition of vagal tonus; whereas in severe hypoxia, other accelerator influences are so prominent that it becomes impossible to demonstrate the influence related to reduced vagal tonus. Partial inhibition of these responses by sympathectomy (T_1-T_5) indicates that activity in cardioaccelerator nerves contributes to the heart rate responses. A severe reduction of the accelerator responses occurs in dogs with inactivated adrenal glands and inactivated cardiac neural influences. These results suggest that liberation of catecholamines from the adrenals complements other cardioaccelerator influences during hypoxia and after cyanide administration.

Several conclusions can be drawn from the studies cited thus far. The carotid bodies are wholly or partly responsible for the hypertension and increased respiratory minute volume observed during systemic hypoxia. They do not contribute to the cardioaccelerator response and in fact they probably evoke a decrease in heart rate. The aortic bodies may be partly involved in the cardiac accelerator response to hypoxia, as well as in some degree related to the hypertension and hyperventilation; however, the exact pattern of responses elicited by stimulation of the aortic bodies is not consistent. Certainly, the aortic bodies cannot possibly play a major role in severe hypoxia. In fact, if one considers that the carotid bodies cause bradycardia and that the aortic bodies cause tachycardia, then the algebraic summation of these two effects would lead to a negligible heart rate response. Activation of pulmonary stretch-receptor afferent nerves, as well as concomitant hypocapnia associated with the elevated respiratory minute volume, contribute in part to the cardiac accelerator response.

The relative importance of the parasympathetic and sympathetic nervous pathways in the mediation of the cardiac responses to hypoxia has not been clearly defined, although it is justifiable to make two points. First, withdrawal of tonic, vagal inhibitory effects on the heart most likely occurs, and this is more important in the less severe stages of hypoxia. Second, discharge of the sympathetic cardioaccelerator nerves, as well as the release of catecholamines from the adrenal medulla are more important factors, although the relative contribution of each component has not been assessed.

III. INITIATING FACTORS

Alexander (1945) postulated a central basis for the cardiovascular responses to systemic hypoxia. He subjected chloralose-anesthetized cats to cervical and lumbar spinal cord transections. The segments of the cord between the two lesions were deafferented by sectioning the dorsal roots. The carotid sinuses were inactivated and bilateral cervical vagotomy was performed. Action potentials were recorded from the inferior cardiac nerve. Changes in activity recorded by this preparation were considered to be a result of alterations in the tonic activity of the sympathetic outflow to the heart. When Alexander elevated the arterial blood pressure by epinephrine injection or by sudden occlusion of the aorta, a reduction in tonic activity was observed. Release of the aortic clamp did not lead to an immediate increase in activity in the cardiac nerve, as would occur if the reduction in activity was simply due to a pressure effect. Because of this, Alexander postulated that alterations in blood gas tensions were taking place and were responsible for the change in activity. He found that hyperventilation of the animal reduced activity in the inferior cardiac nerve, while asphyxiation and nitrogen ventilation markedly increased activity. Alexander concluded that changes in blood P_{O_2} act directly on spinal cord sympathetic centers and evoke an increase in sympathetic activity in this manner. Alexander did not analyze effects on heart rate as such, and Randall (1965) has submitted that it is not tenable to make interpretations about alterations in tonic sympathetic, cardioaccelerator nerve activity from this type of preparation since a recording from the inferior cardiac nerve represents only a minute fraction of the total number of functionally intact pathways to the heart. Randall believes that this tonic activity alone could not have significantly influenced the heart rate.

On the other hand, Downing et al. (1963) also favor the hypothesis that hypoxia evokes cardiovascular effects by directly stimulating neurons in the central nervous system. They induced hypoxia, hypercapnia, and ischemia in dogs under extracorporeal perfusion. The CNS was perfused through the brachiocephalic artery, and the venous drainage was collected from the superior vena cava. Central hypoxia, hypercapnia, or ischemia elicited a rise in arterial blood pressure, an elevation in heart rate, and an increase in myocardial contractility. The arterial P_{O_2} reduction was equivalent to that observed during ventilation with 5% O_2 in N_2. Downing et al. concluded that severe hypoxia elicits sympathetic discharge by directly stimulating the central nervous system.

DeGeest et al. (1965) performed a similar series of experiments. However, they found that when the carotid bodies were intact, hypoxia confined to cephalic regions led to an initial depression of ventricular contractility, which was subsequently followed by an increased contractile response. After carotid-body denervation, cephalic hypoxia caused only an enhanced ventricular contractile response. DeGeest et al. (1965) also concluded that a large part of the cardiovascular response could be explained by cephalic hypoxia.

Davenport et al. (1947) noted that in unanesthetized dogs with chronic denervation of the peripheral chemoreceptors, hypoxia evoked a sharp rise in pulse rate and respiratory minute volume, which remained at a high level throughout the period of hypoxia. A prompt fall of these parameters to control levels occurred upon return to ventilation with room air. These studies point to a central basis for the cardiovascular reactions to hypoxia.

IV. CARDIOVASCULAR ADJUSTMENTS

Krasney (1970, 1971b) attempted to test the assumption that the neural control mechanisms that are engaged during cyanide hypoxia and arterial hypoxia are similar. Dogs were anesthetized with morphine and chloralose to such a degree that the normoxic heart rate and the vagal tonus approached that of the conscious animal. Cyanide hypoxia and arterial hypoxia were produced while dogs were breathing spontaneously, during open chest artificial ventilation, and following sinoaortic denervation, which eliminated peripheral chemoreceptor activity as well as the baroreceptor input. Sodium cyanide injections (0.3 mg/kg iv) provoked a rise in cardiac output and venous return, as measured by electromagnetic flowmeters. Both heart rate and stroke volume increased. After sinoaortic denervation, cyanide produced a less marked increase in aortic flow, which was attributed to an increase in heart rate, while stroke volume was unchanged. In addition, there was a striking reduction in the venous return response. Hence, it appeared that the responses of the intact animals with regard to cardiac output and venous return were largely dependent upon reflex circulatory influences most likely arising from the carotid and aortic bodies. An analysis of the regional circulatory responses to cyanide in the hindlimb, subclavian, superior mesenteric, external carotid, and vertebral vascular beds indicated that the peripheral response to cyanide has at least two components: a reflex vasoconstriction and a local dilator action. Local blood flow appeared to be altered in response to cyanide, depending on the relative balance of these mechanisms and the interaction between vascular tone and arterial pressure.

In contrast with cyanide hypoxia, arterial hypoxia (Krasney, 1971a) produced a somewhat different response pattern in morphine–chloralose anesthetized dogs. During ventilation of the dogs with 6% O_2 in N_2, there was a rise in aortic blood flow (cardiac output) as measured with the electromagnetic flowmeter. This response appeared to occur irrespective of conditions of ventilation or relative level of chemoreceptor control of the circulation. It was observed that aortic flow was increased in association with increased heart rate in the spontaneously breathing dog, while an increased stroke volume was favored during hypoxia induced under controlled artificial ventilation and after sinoaortic denervation. Superior caval flow was enhanced at the expense of inferior caval flow during hypoxia in the intact animals. This hypoxic redistribution of systemic flow was abolished by chemoreceptor denervation. An analysis of common carotid and superior mesenteric flows indicated that the peripheral vascular response to arterial hypoxia represents both vasoconstrictor and vasodilator components. As with cyanide, local flow appeared to be altered variably during hypoxia, depending on the relative balance of these two mechanisms. Thus, it is apparent in dogs under morphine chloralose anesthesia that there are residual mechanisms that provide for enhanced cardiac performance following inactivation of the peripheral chemoreceptors during either cyanide hypoxia or arterial hypoxia.

Achtel and Downing (1972) further investigated the mechanisms responsible for increasing ventricular contractile performance during hypoxia. Previous studies had demonstrated that isolated carotid-body hypoxia is not associated with an increase in ventricular contractility (Downing *et al.,* 1962). However, Stern and Rapaport (1967) had reported that increased ventricular contractile performance resulted from pharmacologic stimulation of the aortic-body chemoreceptors. Hence, ventricular contractile performance was studied in atropinized cats before and following denervation of the aortic receptors by bilateral vagotomy. Ventricular contractility was measured under conditions of constant aortic pressure, cardiac output, and heart rate. Arterial blood gases and pH were continuously monitored. All cats with arterial hypoxemia (P_{O_2} 27–47 torr), showed an increase in ventricular contractility manifested by an increase in ventricular dP/dt for a given end-diastolic pressure. The responses were unaltered by bilateral vagotomy. Similar findings were obtained in animals with bilateral carotid-body denervation. The increase of ventricular contractility during hypoxia was not significantly less, following adrenalectomy. β-Adrenergic blockade completely abolished these responses. These authors concluded that the increase in ventricular contractility associated with systemic hypoxia cannot be entirely attributed to aortic or carotid chemoreceptor reflex activity. They pointed to the central nervous system as having an important role in these contractile responses.

Since stimulation of structures within the central nervous system has been considered to play an important role in producing the circulatory adjustments to hypoxia, a number of investigators have experimented with conscious animals where anesthesia would not obtund the neural responses. Variable results have been reported.

Horwitz *et al.* (1969) studied the cardiovascular effects of low oxygen atmospheres in conscious and anesthetized dogs. These dogs were instrumented with Doppler ultrasonic flow transducers on the ascending aorta; catheters were inserted in the left and right atria, pulmonary artery, and thoracic aorta. The dogs were exposed for 30 min to atmospheres with ambient oxygen tensions of 85, 70, 55, or 40 torr in an environmental chamber. Hypoxia resulted in a rise in pulmonary artery pressure, a fall in left atrial pressure, tachycardia, and a fall in stroke volume with no change in cardiac output. Subsequently, some of the dogs were studied during pentobarbital anesthesia, and large increases in cardiac output were noted at mild levels of hypoxia, but a decrease in output occurred at a more severe level of hypoxia. Horwitz *et al.* (1969) concluded that marked differences occur in the cardiac responses to hypoxia in the conscious versus the anesthetized state and that the major hemodynamic alterations in conscious, resting dogs are tachycardia and a redistribution of blood flow. This is one of the few studies reporting no change or decrease in cardiac output during hypoxia in conscious dogs. The reasons for this discrepancy are not clear, but it may be pointed out that the room-air heart rates of these dogs were quite high, i.e., greater than 100 beats/min. These heart rates are greater than those normally observed in conscious dogs (around 60–70 beats/min). These high rates may have influenced the results.

In contrast, the only comparative study of the cardiac responses to hypoxia in man and the conscious dog was performed by Kontos *et al.* (1967). The circulatory response to breathing low oxygen gas mixtures for 7 min was examined in 33 experiments on seven unanesthetized, trained dogs previously fitted with a flowmeter probe on the ascending aorta, and in 35 experiments on 26 young, normal human volunteers. In the dog, hypoxia caused tachycardia, an increase in aortic blood flow, hypertension, and hypocapnia. Consistent increases in aortic blood flow in excess of 10% of the resting value did not occur unless the arterial blood P_{O_2} decreased below 30 torr. In man, hypoxia was associated with tachycardia, increases in stroke volume and cardiac output, decreases in systemic vascular resistance and arterial blood P_{O_2}, but there was no change in mean arterial blood pressure. It was concluded that the circulatory response to hypoxia in man, in general, resembled that of the dogs, except that man failed to show an increase in arterial pressure. It was suggested that the hypertensive effect of chemoreceptor stimulation in man is either relatively weak or it is effectively antagonized by other mechanisms. Also, significant circulatory changes occurred at a higher P_{O_2}, and there were greater increments in cardiac output and heart rate in man as compared with the conscious dog. The reasons for these differences were unclear. Hypocapnia had been consistently found in both man and the dog in such experiments. In order to determine what significance these findings have in relation to the circulatory response to hypoxia, the authors cited two previous studies.

In one investigation (Kontos *et al.*, 1965b), the circulatory responses to hypocapnia were studied in 40 anesthetized dogs. Hypocapnia, when induced without a change in ventilation (by withdrawing CO_2 from CO_2–air mixture breathed by hyperventilated animals), caused a slight increase in limb vascular resistance in six dogs and a decrease in one dog. Hypocapnia induced by hyperventilation caused an increase in limb vascular resistance in six dogs and a decrease in four. Following the administration of phenoxybenzamine into the femoral artery, hypocapnia induced by either method invariably caused an increase in limb vascular resistance in eight dogs. These results were thought to demonstrate a direct vasoconstrictor influence of hypocapnia on limb blood vessels. In the intact limb this response may be opposed by vasodilator effects mediated through the nerves. Hypocapnia induced without change in ventilation had no significant effect on cardiac output, systemic vascular resistance, or arterial blood pressure in eight dogs. However, hypocapnia induced in nine dogs by increased ventilation was associated with significant decreases in cardiac output and systemic arterial pressure and a significant increase in systemic vascular resistance. The latter response was attributed to the effects of intermittent positive pressure used to increase ventilation.

The role of hypocapnia in the circulatory responses to acute hypoxia was investigated in 18 healthy men (Richardson *et al.*, 1966). Cardiac output increased by 76%, heart rate increased by 25%, and arterial pressure did not change significantly in nine subjects who breathed 8% O_2 in N_2 for 7–8 min. When sufficient CO_2 was added to the hypoxic gas mixture to raise arterial P_{CO_2} to its control value, the circulatory changes were reduced, but the arterial oxygen tension was raised from 37 torr to 52 torr as a result of increased ventilation. Abolition of hypocapnia without change in arterial oxygen tension, by reducing oxygen concentration from 9% to 7% when CO_2 was added to the inspired gas, produced no change in the circulatory responses to hypoxia in 12 subjects. Thus, it was concluded that hypocapnia does not appear to be responsible for the increase in cardiac output, heart rate, and forearm blood flow, which accompany acute arterial hypoxia.

Yet, this same group (Kontos *et al.*, 1965b) found evidence in favor of hypocapnia contributing to the circulatory response to hypoxia in the anesthetized dog. The main purpose of their study was to investigate the possibility that mechanisms secondary to the increased ventilation may contribute to the circulatory responses to systemic hypoxia. In 14 spontaneously breathing dogs, systemic hypoxia induced by breathing 7.5% O_2 in N_2 increased cardiac output, heart rate, mean arterial pressure, and femoral arterial flow; however, it decreased systemic and hindlimb vascular resistances. In 14 dogs whose ventilation was kept constant by means of a respiratory pump and intravenous decamethonium, systemic hypoxia did not change cardiac output, femoral arterial flow, or limb vascular resistance; but it significantly decreased heart rate and significantly raised systemic vascular resistance. In seven spontaneously breathing dogs, arterial blood P_{CO_2} was maintained at the control level during systemic hypoxia. The increase in heart rate was significantly less pronounced, but the other circulatory responses were not significantly different from those found during hypocapnic hypoxia. Thus, this study suggests that mechanisms secondary to increased ventilation contribute significantly to the circulatory responses to systemic hypoxia. Hypocapnia partly accounts for the increased heart rate and the other circulatory responses.

More recently, Bing *et al.* (1969) specifically examined the role of arterial P_{CO_2} in mediating the circulatory response to arterial hypoxia in conscious dogs. Moderate hypoxemia (mean arterial O_2 saturation 58%) was produced in an environmental chamber. Respiratory alkalosis occurred along with tachycardia, but there was no change in cardiac output or systemic arterial or pulmonary arterial pressures. Severe hypoxemia (mean arterial O_2 saturation 34%) with respiratory alkalosis elevated cardiac output, on an average, by 109%, largely due to an increase in stroke volume. Correction of the respiratory alkalosis by inhalation of 4% CO_2 reduced heart rate to control levels, in both groups of dogs, without a further change in cardiac output. Acute respiratory acidosis (10% inspired CO_2) elevated pulmonary arterial pressure in moderately and severely hypoxic dogs but did not otherwise alter circulatory dynamics. It was concluded that severe hypoxemia is required to elevate the cardiac output of awake dogs, and that this elevation is mediated primarily by an increase in stroke volume. Tachycardia during hypoxemia, on the other hand, appeared to be related more to respiratory alkalosis than to hypoxia per se. Unfortunately, two deficiencies are apparent in this study. First, in the severely hypoxic dogs, when CO_2 was added to the inspirate, the arterial P_{O_2} did not decline as much because of the greater ventilatory response in normocapnic hypoxia. Within the range of low arterial oxygen tensions produced in this study, it is likely that only a slight difference (a few torr) in the arterial P_{O_2} produced may markedly influence the circulatory response. Second, the dogs were untrained and catheters were placed acutely, under local anesthesia. Thus, the dogs had higher heart rates than those usually observed in conscious dogs, and this factor may be the reason why the cardiac output response was related more to the stroke volume than to the heart rate increase, as is more commonly observed. From such studies it may be concluded that there is some evidence that hypocapnia and mechanisms secondary to the increase in ventilation may contribute to the circulatory responses to hypoxia.

The nature of the efferent limb of the cardiac responses to hypoxia has been studied in the conscious dog (Kontos and Lower, 1969). This study in particular examined the importance of the β-adrenergic receptors. Unanesthetized dogs, breathing 7% oxygen, exhibited increases in heart rate, cardiac output, and mean arterial blood pressure. The tachycardia and elevated cardiac output were abolished by propranolol. The circulatory response to hypoxia could not be reproduced by intravenous infusions of isoproterenol, epinephrine, or a mixture of isoproterenol and norepinephrine. The effect on the circulatory response to hypoxia, following the administration of a small dose (0.075 mg/kg) of propranolol, was distinctly different from the effect of propranolol on the response to catecholamine infusion. Bilateral adrenalectomy did not modify the response to hypoxia in anesthetized dogs. In dogs with cardiac denervation following cardiac autotransplantation, hypoxia produced increases in heart rate and cardiac output which were markedly reduced by propranolol but not modified by bilateral adrenalectomy. Autotransplanted dogs responded to hypoxia before and after propranolol like the unanesthetized dogs, following cardiac reinnervation. The results suggest that stimulation of cardiac β-adrenergic receptors is a major factor in the production of tachycardia and increased cardiac output during hypoxia. In a normal dog, this is the result of increased activity of cardiac sympathetic nerves rather than circulating catecholamines. In the cardiac denervated dogs, circulating catecholamines are responsible for cardiac β-adrenergic receptor stimulation. This difference between normal and denervated dogs is probably due to the absence of reflex control of the heart and to the hypersensitivity of the denervated heart to catecholamines.

The results of the latter study raise important questions as to the nature of circulatory control during hypoxia in the conscious dog. Browse and Shepherd (1966) have demonstrated that chemoreceptor stimulation can constrict veins. This was examined in dogs by monitoring the changes in venous pressure in a hindlimb where the circulation had been arrested temporarily. The aortic chemoreceptor was stimulated by the injection of 1 mg of cyanide at the aortic valve and by the subsequent stimulation of the carotid body delayed 15–25 sec by the insertion of long tubes (1 m) into the carotid arteries. Repeated stimulation was made during natural breathing, artificial ventilation, and muscle paralysis; after vagotomy with unaided breathing; and after vagotomy with artificial ventilation. The responses from stimulation of both sets of chemoreceptors were similar and were unaffected by the changes in ventilation. Initially, there was a modest venoconstriction which, with repeated stimulation in 6 of 10 dogs, changed to marked venodilation. The response of ventilation and aortic pressure did not change. The venous responses to aortic- and carotid-body stimulation were abolished by vagotomy and sinus nerve division, respectively. Braunwald *et al.* (1963) have additionally demonstrated chemoreflex-mediated venoconstriction.

In addition to this chemoreceptor-mediated venoconstriction, Smith and Crowell (1967) have demonstrated that hypoxia causes a decline in systemic venous capacitance and a consequent elevation of the mean circulatory filling pressure. Hypoxia also causes a drop in the systemic resistance to blood flow suggesting a net systemic vasodilation. These factors, when coupled together, should cause an increase in systemic venous return. An increase in venous return should (on a purely mechanical basis) elevate stroke volume and cardiac output (Guyton *et al.*, 1973). With these relationships in mind, it is difficult to determine why cardiac output did not increase during hypoxia after β-adrenergic blockade in the latter study by Kontos and Lower (1969). If propranolol was only inhibiting beta receptors, one would have predicted that an increased venous return would raise cardiac filling pressure and stroke volume. This suggests that propranolol might have been inhibiting ventricular contractile responses to increased end-diastolic volume, or that β-receptor-mediated venoconstrictor responses were inhibited.

With respect to the afferent mechanisms concerned in cardiovascular control during systemic hypoxia, Krasney (1971b; Krasney *et al.*, 1973) attempted to determine the relative role of the peripheral arterial chemoreceptors in mediating the circulatory responses to both cyanide hypoxia and arterial hypoxia in the conscious dog. Intraaortic injections of NaCN (0.3 mg/kg) were administered to trained, conscious dogs instrumented with electromagnetic flow probes and left atrial and arterial catheters. Cyanide evoked abrupt significant elevations in cardiac output (35.7%), heart rate (58.7%), and arterial blood pressure (14%), while systemic vascular resistance was unchanged. A reflex hyperventilation accompanied these circulatory responses. In order to determine the role of the carotid and aortic bodies in this response, the carotid and aortic depressor nerves were sectioned. Following a recovery period, intraaortic cyanide injections again significantly increased cardiac output (53.9%), heart rate (22.7%), and arterial pressure (27.3%). Systemic vascular resistance fell initially (26%) and subsequently returned to control levels. Recorded ventilation was unchanged. These results are in striking contrast to the prominent reduction in blood pressure and vascular resistance elicited by cyanide in anesthetized, sinoaortic denervated dogs. Hence, chemoreceptor reflexes are not essential for an increase in cardiac output and blood pressure to occur during histotoxic hypoxia in the awake dog. These experiments support the hypothesis that a major site of initiation for these circulatory responses lies outside the sinoaortic reflexogenic zones, probably within the central nervous system.

In a later investigation, the influence of arterial hypoxia on the circulation of the conscious, chronically instrumented dog was studied (Krasney et al., 1973). A mask was used to expose the dogs to arterial hypoxia ($Pa_{O_2} = 24.5$ torr) for a period of 6 min. Hypoxia caused a 79% increase in cardiac output, a 61% rise in heart rate, and a 22% rise in arterial blood pressure. Ventilation increased 323%, causing hypocapnia and an increase in arterial pH. The carotid and aortic depressor nerves were then sectioned, and, after several days of recovery, the effect of hypoxia was again tested. After denervation, similar levels of arterial hypoxia caused a 64% rise in cardiac output, a 23% rise in heart rate, and no change in blood pressure. There was a slight but significant increase in ventilation (20%) along with no appreciable changes in arterial pH or P_{CO_2}. These observations indicated that arterial blood pressure is relatively well maintained during hypoxia in awake dogs after chemoreceptor denervation, in contrast to the marked decrease in blood pressure observed under these conditions in anesthetized dogs. It has been suggested that the chemoreceptors become more powerful in regulating respiration under conditions of anesthesia. From the studies cited thus far, it would also appear that the peripheral chemoreceptors are also more important in regulating the circulation under conditions of anesthesia. As noted in other studies, it appears likely that a large part of the cardiac output response of the intact animal is initiated outside the sinoaortic reflexogenic zones.

Very few studies are available concerning the applicability of the previously described data to man. However, Lugliani et al. (1973) attempted to determine the importance of the carotid bodies in cardiovascular control in man. They investigated eight subjects who had undergone bilateral carotid-body resection (CBR) without baroreceptor denervation for bronchial asthma. Five normal subjects and three asthmatic patients served as controls. The subject breathed air, 12% O_2 in N_2 and 5% CO_2, and 21% O_2 in N_2, while at rest and during cycle ergometer exercise. During hypoxia (Pa_{O_2} = 40 torr), the tachycardia was not affected by CBR; the heart rate increase averaged 15 beats/min during rest and exercise. The systolic, diastolic, and pulse pressures slowly decreased in the CBR subjects, whereas they increased in the control subjects. Following the subjects' return to air breathing, blood pressure decreased in the control group, whereas, it increased in the CBR subjects. In contrast to the altered response of blood pressure in the CBR subjects during hypoxia, the pressor response to hypercapnia was not different in the two groups. It was concluded that, in man, the carotid bodies are essential for normal pressor responses during hypoxia, but not for the tachycardia of hypoxia or the cardiovascular responses to hypercapnia.

Whereas the peripheral chemoreceptors do not appear to be essential for production of the complete cardiovascular response to hypoxia, several studies have indicated that these reflexes are capable of evoking specific cardiac and regional circulatory responses, which may occur in the intact animal but are compensated for in the chemoreceptor denervated animal.

Stern and Rapaport (1967) studied changes in left ventricular performance, stroke volume, and peripheral vascular resistance after combined and separate stimulation of the aortic and carotid chemoreceptors. Selective stimulation of the aortic chemoreceptors produced an immediate increase in myocardial contractility, as judged by the force developed by a strain-gauge arch sewn into the left ventricular myocardium and by changes in the first derivative of the left ventricular pressure. Similar results were seen when heart rate changes were prevented by prior administration of atropine, when changes in ventricular outflow impedance were prevented by previous blockade of the α-adrenergic receptors, and when there was combined chemoreceptor stimulation. β-Adrenergic blockade prevented the increase in myocardial contractility observed after chemoreceptor stimulation. With selective carotid chemoreceptor stimulation, there was no significant change in contractility. Aortic chemoreceptor stimulation increased the heart rate and peripheral vascular resistance, and decreased the stroke volume; carotid chemoreceptor stimulation slowed the heart rate and increased the stroke volume but did not change peripheral vascular resistance. Nicotine was used as the chemoreceptor stimulant, and it is not clear whether or not similar changes would occur if hypoxic blood were to be used as a chemoreceptor stimulant.

By way of comparison, interesting regional reflex vascular responses to stimulation of the peripheral chemoreceptors with nicotine and cyanide were reported by Calvelo *et al.* (1970). Dogs were anesthetized and artificially respired, and an attempt was made to identify the efferent components of the sympathetic system that are activated in different vascular beds. The gracilis muscle and hind paw were isolated and perfused with blood at constant flow. Changes in perfusion pressure reflected changes in total vascular resistance, and changes in small vein pressure reflected changes in venous resistance. The results indicated that stimulation of carotid and aortic chemoreceptors selectively activates efferent, adrenergic constrictor fibers that supply prevenous resistance vessels in the gracilis muscle and venous resistance vessels in the paw. In contrast, there was a dilation of prevenous resistance vessels in the paw caused by activation of efferent, sympathetic dilator fibers and not by withdrawal of sympathetic constrictor tone. The dilation was not mediated through the release of acetylcholine, histamine, or bradykinin, nor through β receptors. Bilateral denervation of the carotid sinus and the carotid body and bilateral vagotomy abolished the reflex responses caused by injections of the chemicals. These responses were not the result of activation of baroreceptors since they were not reproduced during electrical stimulation of the carotid sinus nerve. It was concluded that individual vascular beds and vascular segments may respond differently or in opposite directions to stimulation of the chemoreceptors. The manner in which these reflexes would integrate with the local vasodilating actions of systemic hypoxia is uncertain.

Specific chemoreflex, coronary dilator effects were reported by the same group (Hackett *et al.*, 1972). Dogs were anesthetized and artificially ventilated, and the peripheral chemoreceptors were stimulated with nicotine. The circumflex coronary artery was perfused at constant flow so that changes in perfusion pressure reflected changes in coronary resistance. Practolol, a myocardioselective β-receptor antagonist, and pacing were used to minimize indirect effects of myocardial responses on coronary resistance. Carotid and aortic injections of nicotine produced decreases in coronary perfusion pressure averaging -21 mm Hg and -22 mm Hg, respectively. Decreases produced after carotid and aortic injections of cyanide averaged -8 mm Hg and -17 mm Hg, respectively. These coronary dilator responses were abolished by bilateral vagotomy or atropine. The coronary dilator responses to carotid chemoreceptor stimulation were accompanied by increases in coronary sinus P_{O_2} in five studies and no change in two studies. Carotid sinus nerve stimulation caused abrupt and sustained coronary vasodilation. After vagotomy or administration of atropine, the response to carotid sinus nerve stimulation was no longer abrupt but occurred gradually, suggesting that a component of the reflex response was blocked. These studies indicate that stimulation of chemoreceptors activates a vagal cholinergic vaso-dilator pathway to coronary vessels in the dog. Activation of this path-way appears also to contribute to the reflex coronary responses to stimu-lation of baroreceptors. The relative role of this coronary chemoreflex in regulating coronary blood flow during systemic hypoxia remains to be determined.

Vatner and McRitchie (1975) studied the coronary vasodilator chemo-reflex in conscious chronically instrumented dogs. They examined the interaction between chemoreflexes and the pulmonary inflation reflex by comparing the responses to chemoreflex stimulation (intracarotid injection of nicotine) when ventilation was allowed to increase with those responses when ventilation was controlled. These responses were also compared with those elicited by both forced mechanical and spon-taneous hyperinflation. When the heart rate was constant, intracarotid administered nicotine induced an increase in the depth of respiration, which was followed closely by an increase in late diastolic coronary flow from 48–106 ml/min and a reduction in late diastolic coronary resistance from 1.62–0.78 mm Hg ml/min. After β receptor and cholinergic block-ade, a similar coronary dilation in response to nicotine occurred only when ventilation was allowed to increase. However, when ventilation was controlled, intracarotid administered nicotine increased coronary resistance after combined β receptor and cholinergic blockade. The reflex coronary dilation was not observed after carotid sinus nerve section or after α-receptor blockade. Thus, nicotine stimulation of the carotid chemoreflex results in a striking coronary dilation that has two components. The minor component involves a chemoreflex with its efferent pathway in the vagi. The major component of coronary dilation follows an increase in the depth of respiration, and its efferent compo-nent appears to involve withdrawal of α-constrictor tone. An almost identical period of reflex coronary dilation followed either forced me-chanical or spontaneous hyperinflation in the conscious dog. Thus, there is strong evidence derived from experiments on both conscious and anesthetized dogs that indicates both chemoreflex and lung inflation reflex control of coronary blood flow. Both of these reflexes are engaged during systemic hypoxia.

Erickson and Stone (1972) examined the mechanisms whereby arterial hypoxia (10% and 5% O_2) mediates changes in coronary blood flow and cardiac function in the conscious dog. When the dogs breathed hypoxic gas mixtures through a tracheostomy, both arterial and coronary sinus oxygen tensions were significantly decreased. With 5% O_2, there were significant increases in heart rate (25%), maximum left ventricular dP/dt (39%), left circumflex, coronary artery blood flow (163%), and left ventricular oxygen consumption (52%), which were attenuated by β-adrenergic blockade with propranolol. When electrical pacing was used to keep the ventricular rate constant during hypoxia, there was no significant difference in coronary blood flow before and after β blockade. β-Adrenergic receptor activity in the myocardium participates in the integrated response to hypoxia although it may not cause active vasodilation of the coronary vessels. While chemoreflex control of coronary flow has been demonstrated, the role of this reflex during systemic hypoxia has been difficult to determine.

Perhaps the first study of coronary flow and ventricular dynamics during hypoxia in the conscious dog was described by Wirthlin and Beck (1966). They studied the effects of simulated high altitudes on phasic, coronary artery blood flow; central aortic pressure and flow; and myocardial metabolism in unmedicated Greyhound dogs 1–2 weeks after implantation of sensing devices. The adaptation of coronary flow to hypoxia was mediated through an increase in heart rate, coronary vasodilation, and an increase in mean aortic pressure. Coronary sinus P_{O_2} was found to correlate highly with arterial P_{O_2}. The linear relationship of coronary flow to oxygen use persisted during hypoxia.

Whereas it appears that the peripheral chemoreflexes are less important in providing general hemodynamic support during hypoxia in the conscious dog, the aforementioned studies dealing with chemoreflex influences upon the ventricle and coronary vasculature suggest that the chemoreflexes may contribute in several specific ways to the cardiac adjustments in systemic hypoxia. Hence, Krasney and Koehler (1977) produced arterial hypoxia in 10 conscious, chronically instrumented dogs by allowing them to breathe 7.5% O_2 in N_2 for 10 min. Hypoxia ($Pa_{O_2} = 28$ torr) caused significant increases in coronary blood flow (+196%), left ventricular dP/dt max (+60%), aortic blood flow (+48%), heart rate (+50%), and left ventricular systolic (+12%) and aortic (+10%) pressures. Left ventricular end-diastolic pressure and stroke volume were unchanged, while systemic (−30%) and coronary diastolic (−66%) vascular resistances declined significantly. When equivalent levels of arterial hypoxia were produced after chronic sinoaortic denervation in four of these dogs, the coronary, cardiac, and systemic hemodynamic responses were not significantly different, with the exception that the small arterial pressure response was abolished. Thus, the peripheral chemoreflexes are not essential for the normal coronary vasodilator and cardiac adjustments to occur during hypoxia in the conscious dog. These data also support the hypothesis that a large part of the cardiac adjustments to hypoxia is initiated outside the sinoaortic reflexogenic zones, probably within the central nervous system.

V. SUMMARY AND CONCLUSIONS

The evidence presented herein assigns a less important role to the carotid and aortic chemoreceptors in regulation of circulation during hypoxia in the conscious dog. This is contrary to previous views. In contrast, the central nervous system appears to be the major site of initiation for the chemical transduction and mediation of the neurally mediated circulatory adjustments to hypoxia. Thus, the peripheral chemoreceptors may play a more important role in regulating the circulation during anesthesia and sleep (Guazzi and Freis, 1969), as is the case with the respiratory limb of the reflex.

This viewpoint raises several important questions. The first relates to the unknown mechanism by which the CNS transduces the response to hypoxia. The second relates to the role of this mechanism during long-term hypoxia, i.e., during adaptation to altitude. Most of the studies cited refer to conditions of acute hypoxia. The cardiovascular system undergoes pronounced adaptation during the first several days at high altitude (Levasseur et al., 1976), and the role of the CNS in mediating these responses is unknown. The evidence for this CNS mechanism is derived by a process of exclusion and some direct evidence provided by several studies. Several of the reflex mechanisms described undoubtedly participate in cardiac or peripheral vascular control in the conscious dog. The only relationship that has been demonstrated is that these reflexes are not essential for the full expression of the hypoxemic response. Other mechanisms may compensate for the absence of these reflexes in the conscious sinoaortic denervated animals. Hence, the importance of these reflexes under closed-loop conditions is unclear.

ACKNOWLEDGMENTS

The investigations performed by the authors and cited herein were supported by Research Grants HL-11982, HL-18416, and HL-14414 from the National Heart, Lung, and Blood Institute. R. C. Koehler was a predoctoral trainee supported by Grant 5-T01-GM00341 from the National Institute of General Medical Sciences.

REFERENCES

Achtel, R. A., and Downing, S. E. (1972). Ventricular responses to hypoxemia following chemoreceptor denervation and adrenalectomy. *Am. Heart J.* **84**, 377–386.

Alexander, R. S. (1945). Tonic activity of spinal cardiovascular centers. *Am. J. Physiol.* **143**, 698–708.

Anitchkov, S. V., and Belen'kii, M. L. (1963). "Pharmacology of the Carotid Body Chemoreceptors." Macmillan, New York.

Baugh, C. W., Cornett, R. W., and Hatcher, J. O. (1959). The adrenal gland and the cardiovascular changes in acute anoxic anoxia in dogs. *Circ. Res.* **7**, 513–520.

Bernthal, T., Greene, W., and Revzin, A. M. (1951). Role of carotid chemoreceptors in hypoxic cardiac acceleration. *Proc. Soc. Exp. Biol. Med.* **76**, 121–125.

Bing, O. H. C., Keefe, J. F., Wolk, M. J., Lipana, J. G., McIntyre, K. M., and Levine, H. J. (1969). Cardiovascular responses to hypoxia and varying P_{CO_2} in the awake dog. *J. Appl. Physiol.* **27**, 204–208.

Braunwald, E., Ross, J., Jr., Kahler, R. L., Gaffney, T. E., Goldblatt, A., and Mason, D. T. (1963). Reflex control on the systemic venous bed: effects on venous tone of vasoactive drugs, and of baroreceptor and chemoreceptor stimulation. *Circ. Res.* **12**, 539–550.

Browse, N. L., and Shepherd, J. T. (1966). Response of veins of canine limb to aortic and carotid chemoreceptor stimulation. *Am. J. Physiol.* **210**, 1435–1441.

Calvelo, M. G., Abboud, F. M., Ballard, D. R., and Abdel-Sayed, W. (1970). Reflex vascular responses to stimulation of chemoreceptors with nicotine and cyanide. *Circ. Res.* **27**, 259–276.

Chalmers, J. P., Isbister, J. P., Korner, P. I., and Mok, H. Y. I. (1965). The role of the sympathetic nervous system in the circulatory response of the rabbit to arterial hypoxia. *J. Physiol. (London)* **181**, 175–191.

Comroe, J. H., Jr. (1965). "The Physiology of Respiration." Yearbook Publ., Chicago, Illinois.

Comroe, J. H., Jr., and Mortimer, L. (1964). The respiratory and cardiovascular responses of temporally separated aortic and carotid bodies to cyanide, nicotine, phenyldiguanide, and serotonin. *J. Pharmacol. Exp. Ther.* **146**, 33–41.

Cooper, T. J., Gilbert, J. W., Bloodwell, R. D., and Crout, J. R. (1961). Chronic extrinsic cardiac denervation by regional neural ablation. Description of operation, verification of the denervation and its effects on myocardial catecholamines. *Circ. Res.* **9**, 275–281.

Daly, M. deB., and Scott, M. T. (1960). The role of the chemoreceptors in the cardiovascular responses to systemic hypoxia in the dog. *J. Physiol. (London)* **154**, 6p–7p.

Daly, M. deB., and Scott, M. T. (1963). Effects of changes in respiration on the cardiovascular responses to stimulation of carotid body chemoreceptors. *In* "The Regulation of Human Respiration" (D. C. Cunningham and B. B. Lloyd, eds.), pp. 149–162. Davis, Philadelphia, Pennsylvania.

Daly, M. deB., and Scott, M. T. (1964). The cardiovascular effects of hypoxia in the dog with special reference to the contribution of the carotid body chemoreceptors. *J. Physiol. (London)* **173**, 201–214.

Davenport, H. W., Brewer, C., Chambers, A. H., and Goldschmidt, S. (1947). The respiratory responses of unanesthetized dogs with chronically denervated aortic and carotid chemoreceptors and their causes. *Am. J. Physiol.* **148**, 406–416.

DeGeest, H., Levy, M. N., and Zieske, H. (1965). Reflex effects of cephalic hypoxia, hypercapnia, and ischemia upon ventricular contractility. *Circ. Res.* **17,** 349–358.

Downing, S. E., Remensnyder, T. P., and Mitchell, J. H. (1962). Cardiovascular responses to hypoxic stimualtion of the carotid bodies. *Circ. Res.* **10,** 676–685.

Downing, S. E., Mitchell, J. H., and Wallace, A. G. (1963). Cardiovascular responses to ischemia, hypoxia and hypercapnia of the central nervous system. *Am. J. Physiol.* **204,** 881–887.

Erickson, H. H., and Stone, H. L. (1972). Cardiac beta-adrenergic receptors and coronary hemodynamics in the conscious dog during hypoxic hypoxia. *Aerosp. Med.* **43,** 422–428.

Gesell, R., and Hertzman, A. B. (1928). The regulation of respiration XXIV. A comparison of the effects of mechanical asphyxia with the lungs filled with room air and with oxygen on the hydrogen ion concentration of the cerebrospinal fluid of the dog. *Am. J. Physiol.* **87,** 24–29.

Glick, G., Plauth, W. H., Jr., and Braunwald, E. (1964). Circulatory response to hypoxia in unanesthetized dogs with and without cardiac denervation. *Am. J. Physiol.* **207,** 753–758.

Guazzi, M., and Freis, E. D. (1969). Sino-aortic reflexes and arterial pH, P_{O_2} and P_{CO_2} in wakefulness and sleep. *Am. J. Physiol.* **217,** 1623–1627.

Guyton, A. C., Jones, C. E., and Coleman, T. G. (1973). "Circulatory Physiology: Cardiac Output and Its Regulation." Saunders, Philadelphia, Pennsylvania.

Hackett, J. G., Abboud, F. M., Mark, A. L., Schmid, P. G., and Heistad, D. D. (1972). Coronary vascular responses to stimulation of chemoreceptors and baroreceptors. *Circ. Res.* **31,** 8–17.

Horwitz, L. D., Bishop, V. S., Stone, H. L., and Stegall, H. F. (1969). Cardiovascular effects of low-oxygen atmospheres in conscious and anesthetized dogs. *J. Appl. Physiol.* **27,** 370–373.

Kontos, H. A., and Lower, R. R. (1969). Role of beta-adrenergic receptors in the circulatory response to hypoxia. *Am. J. Physiol.* **217,** 756–763.

Kontos, H. A., Mauck, H. P., Jr., Richardson, D. W., and Patterson, J. L. Jr. (1965a). Mechanisms of circulatory responses to systemic hypoxia in the anesthetized dog. *Am. J. Physiol.* **209,** 397–403.

Kontos, H. A., Mauck, H. P., Jr., Richardson, D. W., and Patterson, J. L., Jr. (1965b), Circulatory responses to hypocapnia in the anesthetized dog. *Am. J. Physiol.* **208,** 139–143.

Kontos, H. A., Levasseur, J. E., Richardson, D. W., Mauck, H. P., Jr., and Patterson, J. L., Jr. (1967). Comparative circulatory responses to systemic hypoxia in man and in unanesthetized dog. *J. Appl. Physiol.* **23,** 381–386.

Kontos, H. A., Vetrovec, G. W., and Richardson, D. W. (1970). Role of carotid chemoreceptors in circulatory response to hypoxia in dogs. *J. Appl. Physiol.* **28,** 561–565.

Korner, P. I. (1959). Circulatory adaptations in hypoxia. *Physiol. Rev.* **39,** 687–730.

Krasney, J. A. (1967). Efferent components of the cardioaccelerator responses to oxygen lack and cyanide. *Am. J. Physiol.* **213,** 1475–1479.

Krasney, J. A. (1970). Effect of sino-aortic denervation on regional circulatory responses to cyanide. *Am. J. Physiol.* **218,** 56–63.

Krasney, J. A. (1971a). Regional circulatory responses to arterial hypoxia in the anesthetized dog. *Am. J. Physiol.* **220,** 699–704.

Krasney, J. A. (1971b). Cardiovascular responses to cyanide in awake sino-aortic denervated dogs. *Am. J. Physiol.* **220,** 1361–1366.

Krasney, J. A., and Koehler, R. C. (1977). Influence of arterial hypoxia on cardiac and

coronary dynamics in the conscious sinoaortic-denervated dog. *J. Appl. Physiol.*
43, 1012–1018.

Krasney, J. A., Magno, M. G., Levitzky, M. G., Koehler, R. C., and Davies, D. G. (1973).
Cardiovascular responses to arterial hypoxia in awake sinoaortic denervated dogs.
J. Appl. Physiol. **35**, 733–738.

Lambertsen, C. J. (1961). Anoxia, altitude and acclimatization. *In* "Medical Physiology"
(V. B. Mountcastle, ed.), pp. 810–835. Mosby, St. Louis, Missouri.

Levasseur, J. E., Kontos, H. A., Richardson, D. W., and Patterson, J. L., Jr. (1976).
Circulatory effects of prolonged hypoxia before and during antihistamine. *J.
Appl. Physiol.* **40**, 549–558.

Lugliani, R., Whipp, B. T., and Wasserman, K. (1973). A role for the carotid body in
cardiovascular control in man. *Chest* **63**, 744–748.

Nahas, G. G., Mathes, G. W., Wargo, J. D. M., and Adams, W. L. (1954). Influence of
acute hypoxia on sympathectomized and adrenalectomized dogs. *Am. J. Physiol.*
177, 13–15.

Randall, W. C. (1965). "Nervous Control of the Heart." Williams & Wilkins, Baltimore,
Maryland.

Richardson, D. W., Kontos, H. A., Shapiro, W., and Patterson, J. L., Jr. (1966). Role
of hypocapnia in the circulatory responses to acute hypoxia in man. *J. Appl.
Physiol.* **21**, 22–26.

Sands, J., and DeGraff, A. C. (1925). Effects of progressive anoxemia on the heart and
circulation. *Am. J. Physiol.* **74**, 416–435.

Smith, E. E., and Crowell, J. W. (1967). Influences of hypoxia on mean circulatory
filling pressure and cardiac output. *Am. J. Physiol.* **212**, 1067–1069.

Stern, S., and Rapaport, E. (1967). Comparison of the reflexes elicited from combined
or separate stimulation of the aortic and carotid chemoreceptors on myocardial
contractility, cardiac output and systemic resistance. *Circ. Res.* **20**, 214–227.

Toyooka, E. T., and Blake, W. D. (1961). Effect of hypoxia on sympathoadrenal activity in dogs with myocardial insufficiency. *Am. J. Physiol.* **201**, 448–450.

Vatner, S. F., and McRitchie, R. T. (1975). Interaction of the chemoreflex and the
pulmonary inflation reflex in the regulation of coronary circulation in conscious
dogs. *Circ. Res.* **37**, 664–673.

Wirthlin, L. B., and Beck, E. P. (1966). Effect of simulated high altitude on left circumflex coronary flow, blood pressure, cardiac output and myocardial metabolism
in the unmedicated Greyhound dog. U.S. Nav. Aerosp. Med. Inst., Bull. No. 965.

7

Pharmacological Aspects of Neural Control of the Circulation

Chung Chinn

I. INTRODUCTION

In recent years, pharmacological approaches to modifying circulation have focused upon the central nervous system as a fruitful area of investigation. This intense interest and effort has resulted from the recognition that a number of clinically useful drugs for the treatment of hypertension have, as their mode of action, an effect upon the central

NEURAL CONTROL OF CIRCULATION

mechanisms of blood pressure control. Thus, clonidine, α-methyldopa, and propranolol are thought to produce their therapeutic effect of lowering the arterial blood pressure by acting on α-adrenergic, β-adrenergic, or other neural mechanisms within the central nervous system. Moreover, since these drugs also produce a variety of behavioral effects, an intriguing possible relationship between alterations in blood pressure control and behavior is suggested.

The current concerted effort in this area is made possible by the recent technical advances in the neurosciences. In addition to the classical procedures of staining for fibers and cells, the histochemical fluorescence procedure developed by Falck et al. (1962) has allowed the mapping of discrete catecholaminergic or tryptaminergic pathways in the mammalian central nervous system. The recent introduction of the retrograde tracer technique, with horseradish peroxidase (HRP) (Kristensson et al., 1971; LaVail and LaVail, 1972) coupled with monoamine oxidase (MAO) staining, has made the identification of central monoaminergic pathways possible (Satoh et al., 1976; Sakumoto et al., 1978). The neurophysiological approach has continued to provide invaluable information regarding neural connections involved in cardiovascular control (Calaresu et al., 1975). The pharmacological approach to studying the brain from its inner surface via the ventriculocisternal system (intraventricular or intracisternal drug injection) introduced by Feldberg (1963) opened up a new era of central nervous system pharmacological research. Today, the procedure of introducing a drug into the ventriculocisternal system of an animal remains the standard procedure for establishing a central site of action of a drug. Obviously, this procedure is somewhat inadequate, since every part of the brain cannot be reached by a drug injected in this manner.

In this chapter the discussion will be concerned with pharmacological aspects of two functional pathways organized within the central nervous system which play roles in cardiovascular control: the "defense" pathway originating in the amygdala, and the depressor pathway involving the anterior hypothalamus. I will discuss some effects of propranolol and diazepam on the hypothalamically evoked circulatory response and will suggest a possible mechanism of action for these agents. I will also review the evidence supporting an effect of clonidine upon α-adrenergic receptors in the depressor pathway.

This chapter is not intended to be exhaustive, but selective. I hope to present an integrated view that has some support from neuroanatomical, neurochemical, physiological, pharmacological, and behavioral data.

II. SYMPATHETIC VASODILATION IN THE DEFENSE REACTION

A. Neural Pathways

The circulatory adjustments that take place when an animal undergoes the behavioral reactions of arousal, aggression, and flight have been extensively studied. These adjustments include an increase in cardiac output and vasoconstriction in high resistance vessels of the renal, mesentery, and cutaneous beds. The outstanding characteristic of the circulatory adjustment is that there is a sympathetically mediated vasodilation in skeletal muscle (Folkow and Uvnäs, 1948; Hilton and Zbrozyna, 1963; Uvnäs, 1966) leading to a redistribution of blood volume to skeletal muscle. In cats, rats, and dogs, this vasodilation is sensitive to atropine blockade and is therefore termed cholinergic.

The physiological and neuroanatomical studies have indicated that this vasodilation in skeletal muscles is mediated via two pathways; one originates in the motor cortex and the other in the amygdala. The pathway that originates in the motor cortex (Eliasson et al., 1951; Lindgren, 1955) has been reexamined recently by Hilton et al. (1975) and found to be noncholinergic. In addition, it was observed that vasodilation did not occur unless the muscle contracted and the behavioral concomitants of the defense reaction did not appear. Thus, this pathway is most likely involved in exercise rather than agonistic behavior. In fact, Smith et al. (1960) showed that diencephalic stimulation in the dog can produce cardiovascular changes that are quite similar to those seen during exercise. Furthermore, Clarke et al. (1968) showed that electrical stimulation of discrete areas of the motor cortex can elicit skeletal muscle vasodilation and movement of the limb. On the other hand, the pathway originating in the amygdala appears to be more intimately involved in the defense reaction (i.e., the circulatory changes are accompanied by agonistic behavior). This appears to follow the ventral amygdalofugal path via the medial forebrain bundle (Hilton and Zbrozyna, 1963) and to either make a synaptic connection in the lateral hypothalamus or pass through it. Neuroanatomical and electrophysiological evidence indicates that there are direct connections between the amygdala and the lateral hypothalamus (Nauta, 1961; Lammers, 1972), but whether or not these connections are involved in the defense reaction is not known. Although the descending course of this pathway traverses the brain stem, the nature of the synaptic connections, if any, is not known.

B. Synaptic Transmission

Very little is known about the chemical nature of the defense pathway originating in the amygdala. The involvement of cholinergic mechanisms in the amygdala and the lateral hypothalamus is supported by the studies of Lewis and Shute (1967) who made use of the acetylcholinesterase (AChE) staining technique to map out cholinergic pathways in the rat brain. These studies indicated that both structures are richly innervated by cholinergic fibers. More recent studies that measure cholinergic "markers" such as choline acetylase (ChAt) activity, AChE activity, receptor binding, synaptosomal uptake of choline, and acetylcholine (ACh) content have all indicated that cholinergic mechanisms play a role in this part of the brain (Storm-Mathisen, 1977; Hoover et al., 1978; Yamamura et al., 1974). Moreover, the direct injection of cholinergic agonists (such as ACh and carbachol) into these structures can produce the behavioral manifestations of the defense reaction in the rat and cat (Allikmets, 1974). However, it is not known whether or not a direct cholinergic connection exists between the amygdaloid nuclear complex and the lateral hypothalamic area.

Similarly, noradrenergic, dopaminergic, and serotoninergic nerve terminals are found to be distributed in the amygdala and hypothalamus, including the lateral hypothalamus (Hokfelt et al., 1978; Lloyd, 1978). But again, no reports of an involvement of any of these neuronal systems in the amygdalofugal pathway to the hypothalamus are available.

In addition to these most considered putative neurotransmitters, recent evidence points to a possible important role of the inhibitory amino acid γ-aminobutyric acid (GABA) in synaptic processes in the central nervous system (Roberts, 1976). Within the hypothalamus and amygdala, GABA meets most of the criteria required of a substance considered to be a neurotransmitter. (Sytinsky et al., 1978). Although the functional role of GABA in the hypothalamus and amygdala is not well understood, there are suggestions that it may be involved in kindling [the phenomenon by which repetitive, intermittent subthreshold intensities of electrical stimulations of the limbic system eventually produce convulsions (Goddard, 1967)], in cardiovascular control, in aggressive behavior (Sytinsky et al., 1978), and in anxiety states (Costa et al., 1975).

The chemical nature of the descending pathway from the diencephalon to the spinal cord is unknown. In the peripheral part of the pathway in sympathetic ganglia, the muscarinic pathway of sympathetic ganglionic transmission is activated when the defense reaction is evoked from the lateral hypothalamus of the anesthetized cat (Brown, 1969). This finding suggests that the muscarinic mode of transmission in sympathetic ganglia described by Eccles and Libet (1961), along with the nicotinic mode, may subserve some function related to the defense reaction. Not only can this pathway be activated by electrical stimulation of the hypothalamic area, but also by the intracerebroventricular injection of ACh in the anesthetized rat (Krstić and Djurkovic, 1978). The resulting pressor response can be abolished by the intracerebroventricular administration of atropine or intravenous administration of methylatropine. Thus, cholinergic activation of central nervous structures (perhaps those of the amygdala and hypothalamus) can in turn activate the muscarinic pathway of sympathetic ganglionic transmission to mediate the circulatory changes of the defense reaction. It might be recalled that intracerebroventricular, intrahypothalamic, or intraamygdalar administration of cholinergic agonists can produce the behavioral manifestations of the defense reaction (Allikmets, 1974).

III. DEPRESSOR PATHWAY INVOLVING THE ANTERIOR HYPOTHALAMUS

The anterior hypothalamus had been known to be involved in cardiovascular regulation ever since Kabat *et al.* (1935) had shown that electrical stimulation of it elicits a cardiodepressor response in the cat. Recent works have demonstrated that this hypothalamic area is involved in baroreceptor reflexes (Manning, 1965; Hilton and Spyer, 1971; Takeuchi and Manning, 1973). Electrical stimulation of a localized area in the anterior hypothalamus and preoptic region produces a pattern of cardiovascular responses that include a decrease in arterial blood pressure, peripheral resistance, and heart rate. These changes are due to a concomitant sympathoinhibition and parasympathetic activation (Hilton and Spyer, 1971) and are identical to the carotid sinus reflex. This anterior hypothalamic component of the carotid sinus reflex appears to be separate from that involving the nucleus tractus solitarius (NTS), site of the primary afferent synapse of the reflex. Discrete bilateral lesions of the anterior hypothalamus reduced the reflex but did not abolish it. It was completely abolished only when both the NTS and anterior hypothalamus were destroyed. Electrophysiological evidence also points to a baroreceptor input to the anterior hypothalamus. Thus, by recording single unit activity from the preoptic depressor area of the cat, Spyer (1972) showed that 15 of the 372 neurons tested consistently increased their firing rate when the intrasinusal pressure was raised, whereas only six showed a decrease. The pathway from the afferents of the carotid sinus to the anterior hypothalamus is not known. However, recent anatomical studies in the rat have demonstrated that the NTS and serotoninergic neurons of the lower brain stem project directly into the anterior hypothalamus (Sakumoto *et al.*, 1978; Ricardo and Koh, 1978). Other neurons that arise in the lower brain stem and project into the anterior hypothalamus are noradrenergic (Sakumoto *et al.*, 1978). In the cat, reciprocal connections between the anterior hypothalamus and raphé nuclei are known to exist (Bobillier *et al.*, 1976; Sakai *et al.*, 1977). An inhibitory role of serotoninergic neurons in the control of sympathetic preganglionic neurons in the cat has been suggested (Neumayr *et al.*, 1974). However, the studies of Chalmers (1976) and co-workers suggest that serotoninergic neurons play an opposite role in cardiovascular control in the rabbit.

IV. NEUROPHARMACOLOGY

A. Antistress Drugs and the Defense Reaction

Since the circulatory and behavioral effects of the defense reaction are provoked by stressful emotional stimuli, and since such stimuli, if persistent, have been implicated as a possible factor in the etiology of hypertension (Charvat *et al.*, 1964; Hallback and Folkow, 1974), it was natural to suggest that agents having the ability to reduce the consequences of stressful stimuli might be useful antihypertensive agents. The benzodiazepines, with diazepam as a prototype, are examples of such drugs. Recently, β-blockers have also been reported to relieve anxiety states in man. Since these agents are clinically useful in the treatment of hypertension, a possible relationship between anxiety states and hypertension is suggested. Although benzodiazepines are not effective antihypertensive drugs, they do reduce the pressor and tachycardiac effects of hypothalamic stimulation in experimental animals (Chai and Wang, 1966; Sigg and Sigg, 1969; Antonaccio and Halley, 1975). The site from which such tachycardic and pressor responses have been elicited generally has been the posterior hypothalamus. Unfortunately, this hypothalamic site is not part of the described defense pathway. In fact, vasoconstriction in skeletal muscles, accompanied by a sharp pressor response, is usually obtained upon electrical stimulation of this site. When the defense reaction is evoked by stimulation of the perifornical region in the lateral hypothalamus of the chloralose-anesthetized cat, vasodilation in skeletal muscle is attenuated by diazepam in a dose range of 0.1–1.0 mg/kg. As seen in Fig. 1, intravenous administration of diazepam abolished the vasodilation in hindlimb skeletal muscle evoked by electrical stimulation of the perifornical region of the lateral hypothalamus. Although a com-

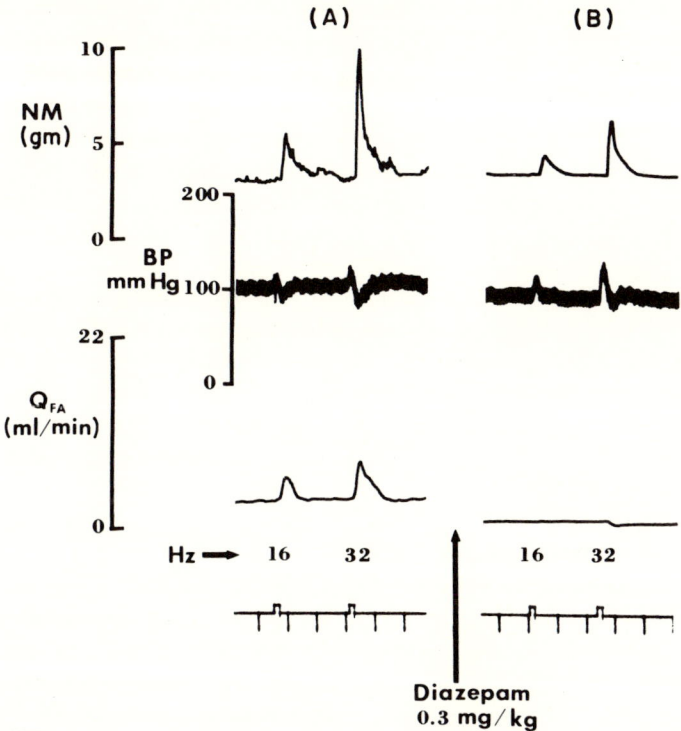

Fig. 1. The effects of diazepam on hypothalamically evoked sympathetic responses in the chloralose-anestheized cat. Panel A: control responses of the ipsilateral nictitating membrane (NM), femoral arterial blood pressure (BP), and ipsilateral femoral arterial blood flow (Q_{FA}) to electrical stimulation of the perifornical region of the lateral hypothalamus (AP = 12.0, Lat = 2.5, HV = 3.0). Stimulation parameters were 100 μA and 1.0 msec duration for 10 sec. Panel B: effects of electrical stimulation 10 min after intravenous administration of diazepam. Femoral arterial flow was measured with an electromagnetic flow transducer.

plete blockade of the vasodilation was seen in this cat, diazepam was usually not as effective in antagonizing the evoked sympathetic cholinergic vasodilation at higher frequencies of stimulation (32 and 64 Hz) as it was at a lower frequency of stimulation (16 Hz) (Chinn and Barnes, 1978). This observation may explain why Bolme *et al.* (1967) did not find an inhibitory effect of chlordiazepoxide, an agent having similar chemical and pharmacological properties as diazepam, on the vasodilation evoked by high-frequency (80 Hz) hypothalamic stimulation of the dog. The inhibition of the vasodilation appears to be of central origin since diazepam is not known to produce a peripheral autonomic effect.

A similar central effect of *dl*-propranolol was also seen since intra-cerebroventricular injection, as well as intravenous injection, produced it. Such an effect is illustrated in Fig. 2, whereby the effects of two doses of *dl*-propranolol were tested on the responses of hypothalamically evoked sympathetic vasodilation, increases in blood pressure, and nictitating membrane tension.

B. Mechanism of Action of Diazepam

Recent ideas regarding the mode of action of benzodiazepines in the nervous system have linked it to an interaction with GABA-ergic neurons (Costa *et al.*, 1975). A variety of biochemical, pharmacological, and physiological observations suggests that the effects of diazepam, the best known of the benzodiazepines, may involve GABA receptors. For example, diazepam is very effective in counteracting the convulsions produced by agents which block the synthesis of GABA (Haefely *et al.*, 1975; Costa *et al.*, 1975). Similarly, diazepam is an effective antidote against the convulsions produced by picrotoxin and bicuculline, two well-known GABA antagonists (Straughan *et al.*, 1971; DeGroat *et al.*, 1972). A variety of neurophysiological evidence provides further support for a GABA-mimetic action of diazepam. Enhancement of presynaptic and postsynaptic inhibition in the cuneate nucleus by intravenous diazepam has been shown by Polc and Haefely (1976). Such inhibitory effects are thought to be mediated by a GABA mechanism, since, when applied iontophoretically, GABA inhibits activity of cuneate neurons (Galindo *et al.*, 1967); whereas, the GABA antagonists picrotoxin and bicuculline block presynaptic inhibition when given intravenously (Banna and Jabbur, 1969; Boyd *et al.*, 1966; Davidson and Reisine, 1971) or iontophoretically (Kelly and Renaud, 1973). When diazepam is iontophoresed onto cuneate neurons, it produces an effect similar to that of GABA (Polzin and Barnes, 1979). Similarly, presynaptic inhibition in the cat spinal cord has been shown to be either enhanced by intravenous diazepam or antagonized by picrotoxin (Schmidt *et al.*, 1967; Ngai *et al.*, 1966; Stratten and Barnes, 1968, 1971; Polzin and Barnes, 1976).

Very recently, a similar GABA-mimetic action of diazepam has been implicated in the action of this drug on hypothalamically evoked cardio-vascular responses in the anesthetized cat (Antonaccio *et al.*, 1978). More interestingly, muscimol and other GABA agonists have been shown to possess a centrally mediated, antihypertensive effect in the anesthetized cat (Sweet *et al.*, 1979). In addition, these authors found that GABA

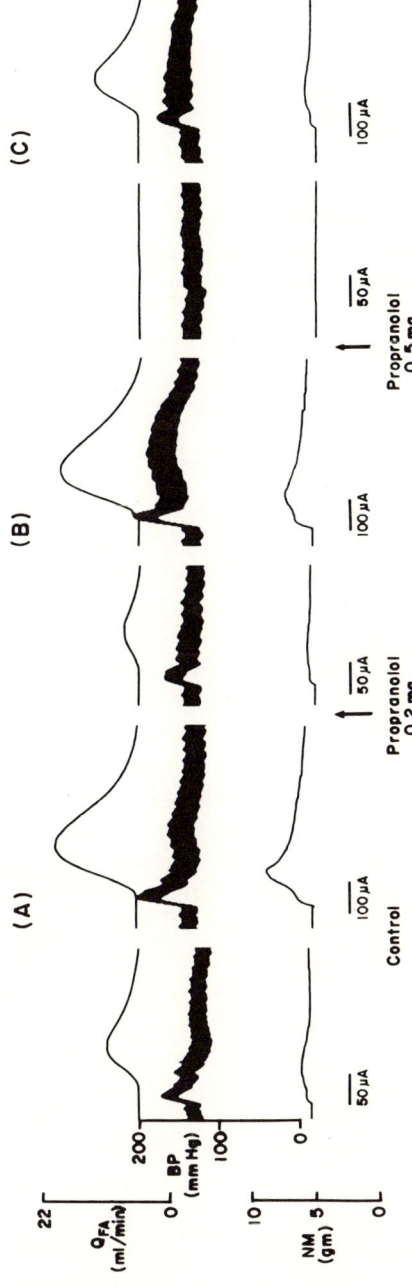

Fig. 2. The effects of propranolol on hypothalamically evoked sympathetic responses in the chloralose-anesthetized cat. Panel A: control responses of ipsilateral, femoral arterial blood flow (Q_{FA}); femoral arterial blood pressure (BP); and ipsilateral nictitating membrane tension (NM) to electrical stimulation of the perifornical region of the lateral hypothalamus (AP = 12.0, Lat = 2.5–3.0, HV = 3–4). Stimulation parameters were 50 μA or 100 μA, 1.0 msec, 100 Hz for 10 sec (indicated by the bar). Panel B: responses 10 min after administration of 0.2 mg dl-propranolol into the lateral cerebroventricle. Panel C: responses 10 min after 0.5 mg dl-propranolol was administered intracerebroventricularly. This second dose was given after responses had recovered from the initial dose.

agonists and analogues can attenuate the baroreceptor reflex via an action on the central components of the reflex.

C. Mechanism of Action of Propranolol

The peripheral β-blocking effect of propranolol is well known; however, the mode of action of this compound in producing a variety of central nervous system effects is a matter of debate. That propranolol can produce central nervous system effects is incontrovertible; however, whether the hypotensive effect is a result of the drug's action on the central nervous system or the peripheral nervous system, or whether β-receptor blockade can explain the hypotension are still controversial questions.

Prichard (1964) originally reported the use of the β-blocker pronetholol in the treatment of hypertension. He believed, along with his colleagues, (Prichard *et al.*, 1977) that propranolol exerts its hypotensive effect in humans via peripheral blockade of β-receptors. Such a belief was based on two findings: (1) that the *d*-isomer of propranolol which has no β-blocking property is also devoid of a hypotensive effect (Waal-Manning, 1970; Prichard, 1970); and (2) that practolol, another β-blocker, possesses a hypotensive effect in humans; but studies in the rat showed that it does not cross the blood–brain barrier (Scales and Cosgrove, 1970).

On the other hand, a variety of observations support a central action of propranolol. Thus, intracerebroventricular administration of propranolol in the anesthetized dog (Srivastava *et al.*, 1973) or the conscious cat (Day and Roach, 1976) results in hypotension. In the conscious cat, the effect appears to be mediated by β-blockade since only *l*-propranolol was active. However, in the anesthetized cat, Kelliher and Buckley (1970) found that both the *d*- and *l*-isomers produced hypotensive effects when administered into the lateral ventricle. Since only the *l*-isomer has the β-blocking property, it was suggested that the hypotensive effect was due to a nonspecific action (local anesthetic) of propranolol. Such a nonspecific action of propranolol, accompanied by a hypotensive effect, was recently demonstrated when the drug was applied to the ventral surface of the brain stem (Bousquet *et al.*, 1978).

However, Lewis (1976) and Day and Roach (1976) have argued strongly for a central β-blockade for the hypotensive effect of propranolol. In support of this position, they have cited the following observations which argue against a peripheral mechanism of action. The major peripheral action of propranolol is a β-blockade on the heart resulting in a decrease in cardiac output and heart rate. These effects occur soon after intravenous administration, with no corresponding decrease in blood pressure (Ulrych *et al.*, 1968). A prolonged decrease in blood pressure occurs later and is due to a decrease in peripheral resistance (Tarazi and Dustan, 1972). Finally, a β-blocking effect of propranolol on vessels would result in vasoconstriction, an effect opposite to the observed one. A renin suppressant effect has also been proposed to explain the hypotensive effect, but the evidence does not support it.

For example, in man, both renin and plasma angiotensin levels return to normal after blood pressure has been lowered by propranolol (Jose *et al.*, 1970; Crane *et al.*, 1972).

That propranolol can exert an effect on the central nervous system to decrease sympathetic outflow, which in turn results in hypotension, was clearly demonstrated by Lewis (1976). By recording blood pressure and preganglionic nerve activity in the splanchnic nerve of the conscious rabbit, they have been able to show that intracerebroventricular administration of *l*-propranolol produces an initial increase in blood pressure accompanied by an increase in nerve activity. This initial effect is then followed by a prolonged hypotension and a marked reduction in nerve activity. Intravenous infusion of propranolol produces only the secondary hypotension and a decrease in nerve activity. These observations clearly point to a central effect of propranolol. How these observations may be related to the clinical hypotensive effect is not clear.

The central β-blockade hypothesis, however, is not without its difficulties. In addition to having to explain the hypotensive effects of *d*-propranolol, which lacks significant β-blocking properties, as described by Kelliher and Buckley (1970) and Klevans *et al.* (1976) in the anesthetized cat; the hypothesis must account for the recent finding by Sweet and Wenger (1976), which showed that lateral ventricular administration of *dl*-propranolol in the unanesthetized, spontaneously hypertensive rat resulted in hypotension only 24 hr after injection. This effect, can not be due to β-adrenergic blockade or to a local anesthetic effect since procaine was administered in a similar way and produced a hypotension that lasted only the first three hours (Sweet and Wenger, 1976).

Finally, a peripheral site of action of propranolol, in the production of its anti-hypertensive effect, was indicated by the studies of Smits and Struyker-Boudier (1979) and Struyker-Boudier *et al.* (1979) in the spontaneously hypertensive rat. In these studies, steady-state concentrations of ³H-labeled propranolol in blood, brain, and other tissues were achieved either by chronic subcutaneous infusions of propranolol or in a lateral cerebral ventricle, by means of the Alzet osmotic minipump. Struyker-Boudier *et al.* found that the hypotensive effect of propranolol was better correlated with peripheral concentrations rather than with brain concentrations of the drug.

Are there hitherto unrecognized properties of propranolol which may produce the clinically observed hypotensive effect? There is evidence from animal studies as well as clinical observations which suggest a similarity of action between propranolol and diazepam. Propranolol possesses anticonvulsant activity (Leszkovszky and Tardos, 1965; Singh *et al.*, 1971; Saelens *et al.*, 1977). Significantly, as found for diazepam (Costa *et al.*, 1975), it is a more effective anticonvulsant against seizures induced by pentylenetetrazole than those elicited by strychnine, a glycine antagonist. Unfortunately, no data of its effects on seizures induced by the GABA antagonists, picrotoxin or bicuculline, are available. A tranquilizing effect of propranolol in rats, which had been made hyperreactive by septal lesions, was reported by Brainbridge and Greenwood (1971). Aggressive behavior of mice induced by isolation was reportedly attenuated by propranolol (Valzelli *et al.*, 1967). In man, propranolol has been known to produce sedation, fatigue, depression, and sleep disturbances (Jefferson, 1974); and it has been effective in the treatment for tremors of Parkinsonism (Owen and Marsden, 1965) and also in treating anxiety (Granville-Grossman and Turner, 1966).

D.   Mechanism of Action of Clonidine

The discovery of clonidine as an effective antihypertensive agent has prompted a large number of studies aimed at localizing its site of action and understanding its mechanism of action. Recent reviews of such studies have been published (van Zwieten, 1973; Schmitt, 1977; Kobinger, 1978). In the cat and rat, clonidine stimulates peripheral and central postsynaptic α-adrenergic receptors (Kobinger, 1978). Since consideration of the peripheral actions of clonidine, including the activation of α-adrenergic receptors, could not account for its potent hypotensive effect, a central site of action was indicated. The following sets of evidence provide strong support for the view of a central site of action. Intracisternal injections of small doses of clonidine produced a decrease in blood pressure and heart rate in anesthetized cats (Kobinger, 1967) and dogs (Onesti *et al.*, 1971). When the same doses of clonidine were given intravenously, the effects were absent or significantly less. Other studies employing intracisternal or intraventricular injections in normotensive animals (Schmitt and Schmitt, 1969; Onesti *et al.*, 1971; Dollery and Reid, 1973) and hypertensive animals (Schmitt and Schmitt, 1969; Reid *et al.*, 1973) yielded similar results. Spontaneous or evoked neural discharges in the preganglionic sympathetic nerves (cervical sympathetic, splanchnic, renal, and cardiac) of cats, dogs, and rats are reduced or abolished by intravenous, intracisternal, or intracerebroventricular administration of clonidine (see Schmitt, 1977). Finally, clonidine facilitates reflex bradycardia in anesthetized or conscious dogs (Robson and Kaplan, 1969; Kobinger and Walland, 1971).

Transection experiments have further localized the central site to be in the medulla of the brain stem (Hukuhara *et al.*, 1968; Schmitt and Schmitt, 1969; Klupp *et al.*, 1970). Various areas within the medulla have been suggested as important sites for clonidine's depressor and bradycardic action. The nucleus of the tractus solitarius, site of the primary afferent synapse of the baroreceptor reflex (Humphrey, 1967; Miura and Reis, 1969), was suggested by Walland *et al.* (1974), Kobinger (1978), and Schmitt (1977) since localized injections of the α-agonist into the cat produced all of the effects of clonidine, except for the initial pressor response. However, more recent studies showed that the central effects of the drug can still be obtained after the NTS has been lesioned (Laubie *et al.*, 1976; Antonaccio and Halley, 1977). The ventral surface of the lower brain stem has also been shown to be sensitive to clonidine (Bousquet and Guertzenstein, 1973). Very recently, Chan and Koo (1978) have localized an area in the medial medullary reticular formation of the rat, which appears to be necessary for the effects of clonidine to be seen. Similar results have been observed in the cat (Chen and Chan, 1978).

A spinal level of action has been proposed by a number of investigators since sympathetic depression has been observed in spinal animals (Sinha *et al.*, 1973; Koss, 1976; Dhawan *et al.*, 1975; Franz *et al.*, 1978).

In addition to the medulla, the anterior hypothalamus has also been found to be sensitive to the direct microinjection of clonidine (Struyker-Boudier *et al.*, 1974). The effects of such a microinjection are like those of the activation of the baroreceptor reflex, i.e., a sympathoinhibition and vagal activation. The result is a slowing of the heart rate and a prolonged hypotension. The importance of the anterior hypothalamus in mediation of the clonidine effects has largely been ignored because in midbrain-transected animals all of the essential cardiovascular and sympathoinhibitory effects of clonidine are seen, as in intact animals with the same doses of clonidine (Schmitt and Schmitt, 1969; Kobinger and Pichler, 1975). In view of the demonstration by Hilton and Spyer (1971) of the participation of the anterior hypothalamus in the baroreceptor reflex, this part of the brain might play an important role in mediating the clinical effects of clonidine.

The similarity of cardiovascular effects to the microinjections of norepinephrine and clonidine to those of the anterior hypothalamus-preoptic region indicates that a similar site and mechanism of action for clonidine and exogenous norepinephrine exists. The effects are mediated by α-receptors since localized prior injections of phentolamine and other α-blocking agents abolish the depressor and bradycardic effects induced by norepinephrine and clonidine (Struyker-Boudier *et al.*, 1974; van Zwieten, 1973). Moreover, the cardiodepressor response evoked by electrical stimulation of the anterior hypothalamus can also be inhibited by push–pull perfusion of the identical area with α-blocking agents in the anesthetized cat (Philippu and Schartner, 1976). Thus, the evidence is quite convincing that α-adrenergic stimulation within the anterior hypothalamic-preoptic area of the rat and cat simulates activation of the carotid sinus reflex. The evidence thus suggests that α-adrenergic stimulation by endogenous norepinephrine, released from noradrenergic nerve terminals within the anterior hypothalamus, partially mediates the cardiovascular responses of the carotid sinus reflex in the rat and cat. Such a role of endogenous norepinephrine in the regulation of the baroreceptor reflex is reminiscent of its role in temperature regulation demonstrated in the cat. Thus, when administered into the cat's lateral ventricle, norepinephrine produced a hypothermia (Feldberg and Myers, 1964). Similar effects were seen when the catecholamine was microinjected into the anterior hypothalamus of the cat (Rudy and Wolf, 1971). The effect was prevented by the prior injection of the α-adrenergic blocker, phentolamine (Rudy and Wolf, 1971). After the cat was warmed, an enhanced release of norepinephrine within the anterior hypothalamus-preoptic area was found to result during the period when the cat attempted to lose heat (Myers and Chinn, 1973). Such an enhanced release of norepinephrine within this brain region might also be expected to occur when the carotid sinus reflex is activated.

V. CONCLUSIONS

The recent discovery of the antihypertensive efficacy of clonidine and propranolol has stimulated much interest in and spurred much research on the question of how these and other centrally active pharmacological agents act on blood-pressure-regulating mechanisms within the central nervous system. In spite of such efforts, there still is no agreement as to how either one of these agents produces its therapeutic effect.

In this perhaps biased and oversimplified consideration of the modes of action of propranolol and clonidine, emphasis was given to two well-known functional systems described in the cat and other species. The so called "defense reaction," in which emotional behavior is integrated with autonomic and somatic systems to achieve a specific physiological function, has received a great deal of attention in recent years. One reason for such interest has been the suggestion that persistent activation of this reaction might produce hypertension (Charvat *et al.,* 1964; Hilton, 1965, 1977; Folkow and Neil, 1971). Direct evidence derived from experimental or clinical studies are lacking to enable us to deny or support this supposition. It may be because of this state of affairs that little effort has been expended to examine the pharmacological aspects of the defense reaction and hypertension. Moreover, diazepam, which effectively abolishes the behavioral as well as the cardiovascular effects of the defense reaction, is not known to be a useful hypotensive agent.

In view of the recent hypothesis that the action of diazepam may be mediated by GABA receptors and that GABA may play a role in controlling the behavioral and cardiovascular changes of the defense reaction, it would appear worthwhile to reexamine the question employing diazepam and other GABA-mimetic agents. Experimental studies and clinical observations suggesting that propranolol has certain similar pharmacological properties as diazepam provide a further basis for pursuing the question.

As for the mechanism of action of clonidine, an action on the α-adrenergic receptor within the anterior hypothalamus is almost a certainty. Facilitation of the carotid sinus reflex, as well as activation of responses similar to those of the carotid sinus reflex, suggest the anterior hypothalamus as a likely site to mediate the cardiovascular effects since the effects of clonidine can still be obtained after NTS lesion. The importance of this action on the carotid sinus reflex, involving the anterior hypothalamus in clonidine-induced hypotension, remains to be demonstrated.

ACKNOWLEDGMENT

The data reported herein and the writing of this chapter was partially supported by NIH Grant HL07789, awarded to Charles D. Barnes.

REFERENCES

Allikmets, L. H. (1974). Cholinergic mechanisms in aggressive behavior. *Med. Biol.* **52,** 19–30.

Antonaccio, M. J., and Halley, J. (1975). Inhibition of centrally evoked pressor responses by diazepam: evidence for an exclusively supramedullary action. *Neuropharmacology* **14,** 649–657.

Antonaccio, M. J., and Halley, J. (1977). Clonidine hypotension: Lack of effect of bilateral lesions of the nucleus solitary tract in anesthetized cats. *Neuropharmacology* **16,** 431–433.

Antonaccio, M. J., Kerwin, L., and Taylor, D. G. (1978). Effects of central GABA receptor agonism and antagonism on evoked diencephalic cardiovascular responses. *Neuropharmacology* **17**, 597–603.

Bainbridge, J. G., and Greenwood, D. T. (1971). Tranquillizing effects of propranolol demonstrated in rats. *Neuropharmacology* **10**, 453–458.

Banna, N. R., and Jabbur, S. J. (1969). Pharmacological studies on inhibition in the cuneate nucleus of the cat. *Int. J. Neuropharmacol.* **8**, 299–307.

Bobillier, P., Seguin, S., Petitjean, F., Salvert, D., Touret, M., and Jouvet, M. (1976). The raphe nuclei of the cat brain stem: a topographical atlas of their efferent projections as revealed by autoradiography, *Brain Res.* **113**, 449–486.

Bolme, P., Ngai, S. H., Uvnas, B., and Wallenberger, L. R. (1967). Circulatory and behavioral effects on electrical stimulation of the sympathetic vasodilator areas in the hypothalamus and mesencephalon in unanesthetized dogs. *Acta Physiol. Scand.* **70**, 334–346.

Bousquet, P., and Guertzenstein, P. G. (1973). Localization of the central cardiovascular action of clonidine. *Br. J. Pharmacol.* **49**, 573–579.

Bousquet, P., Feldman, J., Bloch, R., and Schwartz, J. (1978). Is the hypotensive effect obtained by application of drugs to the ventral surface of the brain stem due to a membrane stabilizing mechanism? A study with beta-blockers. *Neuropharmacology* **17**, 605–609.

Boyd, E. S., Meritt, D. A., and Gardner, L. C. (1966). The effect of convulsant drugs on transmission through the cuneate nucleus. *J. Pharmacol. Exp. Ther.* **154**, 398–409.

Brown, A. M. (1969). Sympathetic ganglionic transmission and the cardiovascular changes of the defense reaction in the cat. *Cir. Res.* **24**, 843–849.

Calaresu, F. R., Faiers, A. A., and Mogenson, G. J. (1975). Central neural regulation of heart and blood vessels in mammals. *Prog. Neurobiol.* **5**, 1–35.

Chai, C. Y., and Wang, S. C. (1966). Cardiovascular actions of diazepam in the cat. *J. Pharmacol. Exp. Ther.* **154**, 271–280.

Chalmers, J. P. (1976). Neuropharmacology of central mechanisms regulating pressure. *In* "Central Actions of Drugs in Blood Pressure Regulation" (J. L. Reid and D. S. Davies, eds.), pp. 36–60. Univ. Park Press, Baltimore, Maryland.

Chan, S. H. H., and Koo, A. (1978). The participation of medullary reticular formation in clonidine-induced hypotension in rats. *Neuropharmacology* **17**, 367–373.

Charvat, J., Dell, P., and Folkow, B. (1964). Mental factors and cardiovascular disease. *Cardiologica* **44**, 124–141.

Chen, Y. H., and Chan, S. H. H. (1978). Clonidine-induced hypotension and bradycardia in cats: the role of medial medullary reticular α-adrenoceptors and vagus nerve. *Soc. Neurosci. Abstr.* **4**, 47.

Chinn, C., and Barnes, C. D. (1978). Comparative effects of propranolol and diazepam on hypothalamically-evoked sympathetic responses. *Pharmacologist* **20**, 207. (Abstr.)

Clarke, N. P., Smith, O. A., and Shearn, D. W. (1968). Topographical representation of vascular smooth muscle of limbs in the primate motor cortex. *Am. J. Physiol.* **214**, 122–129.

Costa, E., Guidotti, A., Mao, C. C., and Suria, A. (1975). New concepts on the mechanism of action of benzodiazepines. *Life Sci.* **17**, 167–186.

Crane, M. G., Harris, J. J., and Johns, V. J. (1972). Hyporeninemic hypertension. *Am. J. Med.* **52**, 457–466.

Davidson, N., and Reisine, H. (1971). Presynaptic inhibition in cuneate blocked by GABA antagonists. *Nature (London) New Biol.* **234**, 223–224.

Day, M. D., and Roach, A. G. (1976). Centrally mediated cardiovascular effects of propranolol and other β-adrenoceptor antagonists in the conscious cat. *In* "Central Action of Drugs in Blood Pressure Regulation" (J. L. Reid and D. Davies, eds.), pp. 215–224. Univ. Park Press, Baltimore, Maryland.

DeGroat, W. C., Lalley, P. M., and Saum, W. R. (1972). Depolarization of dorsal root ganglia in the cat by GABA and related amino acids: Antagonism by picrotoxin and bicuculline. *Brain Res.* **44**, 273–277.

Dhawan, B. N., Johri, M. B., Singh, G. B., Srimal, R. C., and Viswesaram, D. (1975). Effect of clonidine on the excitability of vasomotor loci in the cat. *Br. J. Pharmacol.* **54**, 17–21.

Dollery, C. T., and Reid, J. L. (1973). Central noradrenergic neurones and the cardiovascular actions of clonidine in the rabbit. *Br. J. Pharmacol.* **47**, 206–216.

Eccles, R. M., and Libet, B. (1961). Origin and blockage of the synaptic responses of curarized sympathetic ganglia. *J. Physiol. (London)* **157**, 484–503.

Eliasson, S., Folkow, B., Lindgren, P., and Uvnas, B. (1951). Activation of sympathetic vasodilator nerves to the skeletal muscles in the cat by hypothalamic stimulation. *Acta Physiol. Scand.* **23**, 333–351.

Falck, B., Hillarp, N. A., Thieme, G., and Torp, A. (1962). Fluorescence of catecholamines and related compounds condensed with formaldehyde. *J. Histochem. Cytochem.* **10**, 348–354.

Feldberg, W. (1963). "A Pharmacological Approach to the Brain from its Inner and Outer Surface." Williams & Wilkins, Baltimore, Maryland.

Feldberg, W., and Myers, R. D. (1964). Effects on temperature of amines injected into the cerebral ventricles. A new concept of temperature regulation. *J. Physiol. (London)* **173**, 226–237.

Folkow, B., and Neil, E. (1971). "Circulation." Oxford Univ. Press, London and New York.

Folkow, B., and Uvnäs, B. (1948). The distribution and functional significance of sympathetic vasodilators to the hind limbs of the cat. *Acta Physiol. Scand.* **15**, 389–400.

Franz, D. N., Hare, B. D., and Neumayr, R. J. (1978). Depression of sympathetic preganglionic neurons by clonidine: evidence for stimulation of 5-HT receptors. *Clin. Exp. Hypertension* **1**, 115–140.

Galindo, A., Krnjevic, K., and Schwartz, S. (1967). Micro-iontophorectic studies on neurones in the cuneate nucleus. *J. Physiol. (London)* **192**, 359–377.

Goddard, G. V. (1967). Development of epileptic seizures through brain stimulation at low intensity. *Nature (London)* **214**, 1020–1021.

Granville-Grossman, K. L., and Turner, P. (1966). The effect of propranolol on anxiety. *Lancet* **1**, 788–790.

Haefely, N., Kulcsar, A., Mohler, H., Pieri, L., Polc, P., and Schaffner, R. (1975). Possible involvement of GABA in the central actions of benzodiazepines. *In* "Mechanism of Action of Benzodiazepines" (E. Costa and P. Greengard, eds.), Advances in Biochemical Psychopharmacology, Vol. 14, pp. 131–151. Raven, New York.

Hallback, M., and Folkow, B. (1974). Cardiovascular responses to acute mental "stress" in spontaneously hypertensive rats. *Acta Physiol. Scand.* **90**, 684–698.

Hilton, S. M. (1965). Hypothalamic control of the cardiovascular responses in fear and rage. *Sci. Basis Med. Annu. Rev.* pp. 217–238.

Hilton, S. M. (1975). Ways of viewing the central nervous control of the circulation—old and new. *Brain Res.* **87**, 213–219.

Hilton, S. M. (1977). Supramedullary organization of vasomotor control. *In* "Progress in Brain Research, Hypertension and Brain Mechanisms" (W. deJong and A. P. Provoost, eds.), pp. 77–81. Elsevier, Amsterdam.

Hilton, S. M., and Spyer, K. M. (1971). Participation of the anterior hypothalamus in the baroreceptor reflex. *J. Physiol. (London)* 218, 271–293.

Hilton, S. M., and A. W. Zbrozyna (1963). Amygdaloid region for the defence reactions and its efferent pathway to the brain stem. *J. Physiol. (London)* 165, 160–173.

Hilton, S. M., Spyer, K. M., and Timms, R. J. (1975). Hind limb vasodilation evoked by stimulation of the motor cortex. *J. Physiol. (London)* 252, 22–23.

Hokfelt, T., Elde, R., Fuxe, K., Johansson, O., Ljungdahl, A., Goldstein, M., Luft, R., Efendic, S., Nilsson, G., Terenius, L., Ganten, D., Jeffcoate, S. L., Rehfeld, J., Said, S., de la Mora, M. P., Possani, L., Tapia, R., Teran, L., and Palacios, R. (1978). Aminergic and peptidergic pathways in the nervous system with special reference to the hypothalamus. *In* "The Hypothalamus" (S. Reichlin, R. J. Baldessarinig, and J. B. Martin, eds.), Research Publications, Association for Research in Nervous and Mental Disease, Vol. 56, pp. 69–135. Raven, New York.

Hoover, D. B., Muth, E. A., and Jacobowitz, D. M. (1978). A mapping of the distribution of acetylcholine, choline acetyltransferase and acetylcholinesterase in discrete areas of rat brain. *Brain Res.* 153, 295–306.

Hukuhara, V. T., Jr., Otsuka, Y., Takeda, R., and Sakai, F. (1968). Die zentralen Wirkungen des 2-(2,6 dichlorphenylamino)-2-imidazolin-hydochlorids. *Arzneim.-Forsch.* 18, 1147–1153.

Humphrey, D. R. (1967). Neuronal activity in the medulla oblongata of cat evoked by stimulation of the catotid sinus nerve. *In* "Baroreceptors and Hypertension" (P. Kezdi, ed.), pp. 131–168. Pergamon, Oxford.

Jefferson, J. W. (1974). Beta-adrenergic receptor blocking drugs in psychiatry. *Arch. Gen. Psychiatry* 31, 681–691.

Jose, A., Crout, S. R., and Kaplan, N. M. (1970). Suppressed plasma renin activity in essential hypertension: roles of plasma volume, blood pressure, and sympathetic nervous sytem. *Ann. Intern. Med.* 72, 9–16.

Kabat, H., Magoun, H. W., and Ranson, S. W. (1935). Electrical stimulation of points in the forebrain and midbrain. The resultant alteration in blood pressure. *Arch. Neurol. Psychiatry* 34, 931–955.

Kelliher, G. J., and J. P. Buckley (1970). Central hypotensive activity of dl- and d-propranolol. *J. Pharm. Sci.* 59, 1276–1280.

Kelly, J. S., and Renaud, L. P. (1973). On the pharmacology of ascending, descending, and recurrent postsynaptic inhibition of the cuneothalamic relay cells in the cat. *Br. J. Pharmacol.* 48, 396–408.

Klevans, L. L., Kovacs, J. L., and Kelly, R. (1976). Central effect of beta-adrenergic blocking agents on arterial blood pressure. *J. Pharmacol. Exp. Ther.* 196, 389–395.

Klupp, H., Knappen, F., Otsuka, Y., Streller, J., and Teichmann, H. (1970). Effects of clonidine on central sympathetic tone. *Eur. J. Pharmacol.* 10, 225–229.

Kobinger, N. (1967). Uber den Wirkungsmechanismus einer neuen antihypertensiven Substanz mit Imidazolinstruktur. *Naunyn-Schmiedebergs Arch. Pharmakol. Exp. Pathol.* 258, 48–68.

Kobinger, W. (1978). Central α-adrenergic systems as targets for hypotensive drugs. *Ergeb. Physiol., Biol. Chem. Exp. Pharmackl.* 81, 40–100.

Kobinger, W., and Pichler, L. (1975). Localization in the CNS of adrenoceptors which facilitate a cardioinhibitory reflex. *Naunyn-Schmiedeberg's Arch. Pharmacol.* 286, 371–377.

Kobinger, W., and Walland, A. (1971). Involvement of adrenergic receptors in central vagus activity. *Eur. J. Pharmacol.* **16,** 120–122.

Koss, M. C. (1976). Studies on the site of action of clonidine utilizing a sympathetic-cholinergic system. *Eur. J. Pharmacol.* **37,** 381–384.

Kristensson, K., Olsson, Y., and Sjostrand, J. (1971). Axonal uptake and retrograde transport of exogeneous proteins in the hypoglossal nerve. *Brain Res.* **32,** 399–406.

Krstić, M. K., and Djurkovic, D. (1978). Cardiovascular responses to intracerebroventricular administration of acetylcholine in rats. *Neuropharmacology* **17,** 341–347.

Lammers, H. J. (1972). The neural connections of the amygdaloid complex in mammals. *In* "Neurobiology of the Amygdala" (B. E. Eleftheriou, ed.), pp. 123–144. Plenum, New York.

Laubie, M., Schmitt, H., and Drouillat, M. (1976). Action of clonidine on the baroreceptor pathways and medullary sites mediating vagal bradycardia. *Eur. J. Pharmacol.* **38,** 293–303.

LaVail, J. H., and LaVail, M. M. (1972). Retrograde axonal transport in the central nervous system. *Science* **176,** 1416–1417.

Leszkovszky, G., and Tardos, L. (1965). Some effects of propranolol on the central nervous system. *J. Pharm. Pharmacol.* **17,** 518–519.

Lewis, P. J. (1976). Propanolol—An antihypertensive drug with a central action. *In* "Central Action of Drugs in Blood Pressure Regulation" (D. Davies and J. L. Reid, eds.), pp. 206–214. Univ. Park Press, Baltimore, Maryland.

Lewis, P. R., and Shute, C. C. D. (1967). The cholinergic limbic system: projections to hippocampal formation, medial cortex, nuclei of the ascending cholinergic reticular system, and the subfornical organ and supraoptic crest. *Brain* **90,** 521–540.

Lindgren, P. (1955). The mesencephalon and the vasomotor system. *Acta Physiol. Scand., Suppl.* **121,** 1–189.

Lloyd, K. G. (1978). The biochemical pharmacology of the limbic system: neuroleptic drugs. *In* "Limbic Mechanisms" (K. E. Livingston and O. Hornykiewicz, eds.), pp. 263–305. Plenum, New York.

Manning, J. W. (1965). Cardiovascular reflexes following lesions in medullary reticular formation. *Am. J. Physiol.* **208,** 283–288.

Miura, M., and Reis, D. J. (1969). Termination and secondary projections of carotid sinus nerve in the cat brain stem. *Am. J. Physiol.* **217,** 142–153.

Myers, R. D., and Chinn, C. (1973). Evoked release of hypothalamic norepinephrine during thermoregulation in the cat. *Am. J. Physiol.* **224,** 230–236.

Nauta, W. J. H. (1961). Fibre degeneration following lesions of the amygdaloid complex in the monkey. *J. Anat.* **95,** 515–531.

Neumayr, R. J., Hare, B. D., and Franz, D. N. (1974). Evidence for bulbospinal control of sympathetic preganglionic neurons by monoaminergic pathways. *Life Sci.* **14,** 793–806.

Ngai, S. H., Tseng, D. T. C., and Wang, S. C. (1966). Effect of diazepam and other central nervous system depressants on spinal reflexes in cats: A study of site of action. *J. Pharmacol. Exp. Ther.* **153,** 344–351.

Onesti, G., Schwartz, A. B., Kim, K. E., Part-Martinez, V., and Swartz, C. (1971). Antihypertensive effect of clonidine. *Circ. Res.* **28,** Suppl. 2, 53–69.

Owen, D. A. L., and Marsden, C. D. (1965). Effect of adrenergic β-blockade on Parkinsonian tremor. *Lancet* **2,** 1259–1262.

Philippu, A., and Schartner, P. (1976). Inhibition by locally applied alpha adrenoreceptor blocking drugs of the depressor response to stimulation of the anterior hypothalamus. *Naunyn-Schmiedeberg's Arch. Pharmacol.* **295,** 1–7.

Polc, P., and Haefely, W. (1976). Effects of two benzoiazepines, phenobarbitone and baclofen on synaptic transmission in the cat cuneate nucleus. *Naunyn-Schmiedeberg's Arch. Pharmacol.* **294,** 121–131.

Polzin, R., and C. D. Barnes (1976). The effect of diazepam and picrotoxin on brain stem evoked dorsal root potentials. *Neuropharmacology* **15,** 133–137.

Polzin, R., and Barnes, C. D. (1979). Effect of diazepam on GABAergic cuneate neurons. *Neuropharmacology* **18,** 431–434.

Prichard, B. N. C. (1964). Hypotensive action of pronethalol. *Br. Med. J.* **1,** 1227–1228.

Prichard, B. N. C. (1970). Aspects of the evaluation of antihypertensive drugs. *Proc. Int. Symp. Clin. Pharmacol., R. Acad. Med. Belg., Brussels* p. 193.

Prichard, B. N. C., Conolly, M. E., Shand, D. G., and Oates, J. A. (1977). Beta-adrenoreceptor blocking drugs. *In* "Handbook of Experimental Pharmacology: Antihypertensive Agents" (F. Gross, ed.), Vol. 39, pp. 589–632. Springer-Verlag, Berlin and New York.

Reid, J. L., Briant, R. H., and Dollery, C. T. (1973). Desmethylimipramine and the hypotensive action of clonidine in the rabbit. *Life Sci.* **12,** 459–467.

Ricardo, J. A., and Koh, E. T. (1978). Anatomical evidence of direct projections from the nucleus of the solitary tract to the hypothalamus, amygdala and other forebrain structures in the rat. *Brain Res.* **153,** 1–26.

Roberts, E. (1976). Disinhibition as an organizing principle in the nervous system—The role of the GABA system. Application to neurologic and psychiatric disorders. *In* "GABA in Nervous System Function" (E. Roberts, T. N. Chase, and D. B. Tower, eds.), pp. 515–539. Raven, New York.

Robson, R. D., and Kaplan, H. R. (1969). An involvement of St 155 [2-(2,6-dichlorphenylamino)-2-imidazoline hydrochloride, Catapres)] in cholinergic mechanisms. *Eur. J. Pharmacol.* **5,** 328–337.

Rudy, T. A., and Wolf, H. H. (1971). The effect of intrahypothalamically injected sympathomimetic amines on temperature regulation in the cat. *J. Pharmacol. Exp. Ther.* **179,** 218–235.

Saelens, D. A., Walle, T., Gaffney, T. E., and Privitera, P. J. (1977). Studies on the contribution of active metabolites to the anticonvulsant effects of propranolol. *Eur. J. Pharmacol.* **42,** 39–46.

Sakai, K., Salvert, D., Touret, M., and Jouvet, M. (1977). Afferent connections of the nucleus raphe dorsalis in the cat as visualized by the horseradish peroxidase technique. *Brain Res.* **137,** 11–35.

Sakumoto, T., Tohyama, M., Satoh, K., Kimoto, Y., Kinugasa, T., Tanizawa, O., Kurachi, K. and Shimizu, N. (1978). Afferent fiber connections from lower brain stem to hypothalamus studied by the horseradish peroxidase method with special reference to noradrenaline innervation. *Exp. Brain Res.* **31,** 81–94.

Satoh, K., Yamamoto, K., Sakumoto, T., Tohyama, M., and Shimizu, N. (1976). Combination of HRP-method with Glenner's MAO staining. *Proc. Int. Congr. Histochem. Cytochem.* 304–305.

Scales, B., and Cosgrove, M. B. (1970). The metabolism and distribution of the selective adrenergic beta blocking agent, practolol. *J. Pharmacol. Exp. Ther.* **175,** 338–347.

Schmidt, R. F., Vogel, M. E., and Zimmerman, M. (1967). Die Wirkung von Diazepam auf die prasyaptische Hemmung und andere Ruckenmarks-reflexe. *Naunyn-Schmiedeberg's Arch. Pharmacol.* **258,** 69–82.

Schmitt, H. (1977). The pharmacology of clonidine and related products. *In* "Handbook of Experimental Pharmacology: Antihypertensive Agents" (F. Gross, ed.), Vol. 39, pp. 299–396. Springer-Verlag, Berlin and New York.

Schmitt, H., and Schmitt, H. (1969). Localization of the hypotensive effect of 2-(2-6-dichlorophenylamino)-2-imidazoline hydrochloride (St 155, Catapresan). *Eur. J. Pharmacol.* **6,** 8–12.

Sigg, E. B., and Sigg, T. D. (1969). Hypothalamic stimulation of preganglionic autonomic activity and its modification by chlorpromazine, diazepam and pentobarbital. *Neuropharmacology* **8,** 567–572.

Singh, K. P., Bhandari, D. S., and Mahawar, M. M. (1971). Effects of propranolol (a beta adrenergic blocking agent) on some central nervous system parameters. *Indian J. Med. Res.* **59,** 786–794.

Sinha, J. N., Atkinson, J. M., and Schmitt, H. (1973). Effects of clonidine and 1-DOPA on spontaneous and evoked splanchnic nerve discharges. *Eur. J. Pharmacol.* **24,** 113–119.

Smith, O. A., Rushmer, R. F., and Lasher, E. P. (1960). Similarity of cardiovascular responses to exercise and to diencephalic stimulation. *Am. J. Physiol.* **198,** 1139–1142.

Smits, J. F. M., and H. A. J. Struyker-Boudier (1979). Steady-state disposition of propranolol and its metabolites in the spontaneously hypertensive rat: chronic subcutaneous vs. intracerchroventricular infusion with osmotic minipumps. *J. Pharmacol. Exp. Ther.* **209,** 317–322.

Spyer, K. M. (1972). Baroreceptor sensitive neurones in the anterior hypothalamus of the cat. *J. Physiol. (London)* **224,** 245–257.

Srivastava, R. K., Kulshrestha, V. K., Singh, N., and Bhargava, K. P. (1973). Central cardiovascular effects of intracerebroventricular propranolol. *Eur. J. Pharmacol.* **21,** 222–229.

Storm-Mathisen, J. (1977). Localization of transmitter candidates in the brain: the hippocampal formation as a model. *Prog. Neurobiol.* **8,** 119–181.

Stratten, W. P., and Barnes, C. D. (1968). Spinal effects of diazepam. *Fed. Proc., Fed. Am. Soc. Exp. Biol.* **27,** 571.

Stratten, W. P., and Barnes, C. D. (1971). Diazepam and presynaptic inhibition. *Neuropharmacology* **10,** 685–696.

Straughan, D. W., Neal, M. J., Simmonds, M. A., Collins, G. G. S., and Hill, R. G. (1971). Evaluation of bicuculline as a GABA antagonist. *Nature (London)* **233,** 352.

Struyker-Boudier, H. A. J., Smeets, G. W. M., Brouwer, G. M., and van Rossum, J. M. (1974). Hypothalamic alpha adrenergic receptors in cardiovascular regulation. *Neuropharmacology* **13,** 837–846.

Struyker-Boudier, H. A. J., Smits, J. F. M., and van Essen, H. (1979). Is the central nervous system involved in the long-term cardiovascular actions of propranolol. *Naunyn-Schmiedeberg's Arch. Pharmacol.* **307,** Suppl., p. R45.

Sweet, C. S., and Wenger, H. C. (1976). Central antihypertensive effects of propranolol in the spontaneously hypertensive rat. *Neuropharmacology* **15,** 511–513.

Sweet, C. S., Wenger, H. C., and Gross, D. M. (1979). Central antihypertensive properties of muscimol and related γ-aminobutyric acid agonists and the interaction of muscimol with baroreceptor reflexes. *Can. J. Physiol. Pharmacol.* **57,** 600–605.

Sytinsky, I. A., Soldatenkov, A. T., and Lajtha, A. (1978). Neurochemical basis of the therapeutic effect of γ-aminobutyric acid and its derivatives. *Prog. Neurobiol.* **10,** 89–133.

Takeuchi, T., and Manning, J. W. (1973). Hypothalamic mediation of sinus baro-receptor-evoked muscle cholinergic dilator response. *Am. J. Physiol.* **224,** 1280–1287.

Tarazi, R. C., and Dustan, H. P. (1972). Beta adrenergic blockade in hypertension. *Am. J. Cardiol.* **29,** 633–640.

Ulrych, M., Frohlich, E. D., Dustan, H. P., and Page, I. H. (1968). Immediate hemodynamic effects of beta-adrenergic blockade with propranolol in normotensive and hypertensive men. *Circulation* **37,** 411–416.

Uvnäs, Bfl. (1966). Cholinergic vasodilator nerves. *Fed. Proc., Fed. Am. Soc. Exp. Biol.* **25,** 1618–1622.

Valzelli, L., Giacalone, E., and Garattini, S. (1967). Pharmacological control of aggressive behavior in mice. *Eur. J. Pharmacol.* **2,** 144–146.

van Zwieten, P. A. (1973). The central action of antihypertensive drugs, mediated via central α-receptors. *J. Pharm. Pharmacol.* **25,** 89–95.

Waal-Manning, H. J. (1970). Lack of effect of d-propranolol on blood pressure and pulse rate in hypertensive patients. *Proc. Univ. Otago Med. Sch.* **48,** 80.

Walland, A., Kobinger, W., and Csongrady, A. (1974). Action of clonidine on baroreceptor reflexes in conscious dogs. *Eur. J. Pharmacol.* **26,** 184–190.

Yamamura, H. I., Kuhar, M. J., Greenberg, D., and Snyder, S. H. (1974). Muscarinic cholinergic receptor binding: Regional distribution in monkey brain. *Brain Res.* **66,** 541–546.

Index

E

Eating condition
  cardiovascular response and, 9
  definition, 5
Emotion, cardiovascular response and, 9,
  12, 14
Endorphins, 41–42
Enkephalin, 41–42, 95
Enkephalin-like peptide, in chromaffin
  cells, 104
Epinephrine, 37, 131, 137
Exaggerated reactivity, 82, 90
Exercise, cardiovascular response and, 7–
  13

F

Fastigial nucleus, 33, 34

G

Glutamate, 38–39
Glycine, 38–39
Granule cells, 32–33
Guanethidine, 36

H

Halothane, 87
Heart rate, exercise and, 11–13
Hexamethonium, 36, 106
Histamine, 39–40, 141
Histone kinase, 115
Human, 40, 94, 139–140
6-Hydroxydopamine, 31, 89, 96
Hypertension
  brain and, 82–86
  in man, 94
  sustained, 90
Hypertension, experimental, 82–98
  animal models, 85–86
  in cat, 89–93
  in rat, 87–89
Hypocapnia, 58, 135–137, 140

Hypothalamic defense region, 71
Hypothalamus, 36, 37, 40, 41, 152
  anterior, depressor pathway, 153–154
Hypoxia
  arterial, 123, 132–134
  hypoxic, 123
  neural control of circulation during,
  123–144
  primary tissue, 123
  respiratory and cardiovascular responses
  to, 123–124
  systemic, 123

I

Inferior olive, 33–35
Intermediolateral sympathetic spinal nu-
  cleus, 72, 73
Intermediomedial sympathetic spinal nu-
  cleus, 72, 73
Interpeduncular nucleus, 35
Interpositus nucleus, 33
Intrinsic oscillator theory, 56–58
Isoproterenol, 137
Isorenin–angiotensin system, 40

K

Kindling, 152
Koch curve, 17, 19

L

Lateral funiculus spino-olivo-cerebellar
  pathway, 35
Lateral tegmental field, 28
Lateral vestibular nucleus, 33
Locus coeruleus, 31, 35, 36, 37, 38, 41

M

Mecamylamine, 36
Methylatropine, 153
α-Methyldopa, 25, 82, 150
Monkey, 38–39, 40